This book is a gift to the therapist who works with teenagers – but also to anyone who parents them, teaches them, supports them or has one in their life in some way. Jeanine Connor is a clinician with a deep understanding of her field, who wears her knowledge lightly. She models a way of relating to her young clients (and their parents/carers) that will be an inspiration for others in the field. Perhaps most importantly, she demonstrates how we can enjoy young people, even the most challenging ones, and genuinely help them navigate complex issues at this turbulent life stage.

Graham Music is a consultant psychotherapist at the Tavistock Centre, and author of *Respark* **(2022),** *Nurturing Children* **(2019),** *Nurturing Natures* **(2018) and** *The Good Life* **(2014).**

This is an absolute gem of a book. The nine stories ingeniously weave together a number of key considerations in this type of work: applied theory and theorists; psychoeducation; safeguarding; cultural sensitivity; the careful considerations of contact and boundaries with parents/caregivers, and much more. The book is also packed with useful resource recommendations. What I love most about Connor's writing is the simplicity with which she explains even complex theory; after 25 years doing this work, she knows and models her craft effortlessly. At times messy, touching and funny, this refreshingly honest exploration of a therapist's process, the workings of the teen mind and the power of the therapeutic relationship is certainly one to read. I rarely cry when I read books – I can't even remember the last time – but I did with this one.

Caz Binstead is an integrative therapist working with young people and adults, a supervisor, founder of #traineetalk and co-lead of #TherapistsConnect

This must-read book totally captures the complexity and fascination of working with this wonderful age group. I loved it. The accounts give an insight into those seemingly small (to us) yet hugely significant (to them) changes that young people experience when taking the brave step of giving psychotherapy a go. From start to finish, I was gripped. I recognised the client voices, so many touchstones, so eloquently delivered in the vivid dialogues. I loved the contributions from the parents and carers too – often a missing voice in the therapeutic landscape, but so essential. The page-turning chapters are engaging, honest and courageous. Jeanine's in-depth analyses draw on a range of psychodynamic and related theory to help make sense of what doesn't always make sense to others. This is an essential, eye-opening read for those training to work therapeutically with young people, and it has much to say to experienced practitioners about staying authentic, keeping it real and generally being kind to yourself in moments of self-doubt. Prepare to have your heart in your mouth and laugh out loud at the same time.

Jo Holmes is a person-centred counsellor, previously working in schools, and is BACP's Children, Young People and Families Lead

'Stop f*cking nodding'

and other things 16-year-olds say in therapy

Jeanine Connor

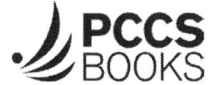

First published 2022

PCCS Books Ltd
Wyastone Business Park
Wyastone Leys
Monmouth
NP25 3SR
UK

Tel +44 (0)1600 891509
contact@pccs-books.co.uk
www.pccs-books.co.uk

© Jeanine Connor

All rights reserved.

No part of this publication may be reproduced, stored in a retrieval system, transmitted or utilised in any form by any means, electronic, mechanical, photocopying or recording or otherwise, without permission in writing from the publishers.

The author has asserted their right to be identified as the author of this work in accordance with the Copyright, Designs and Patents Act 1988.

Stop F*cking Nodding: and other things 16-year-olds say in therapy

British Library Cataloguing in Publication Data.
A catalogue record for this book is available from the British Library

ISBNs   paperback 978 1 915220 08 0
        epub 978 1 915220 09 7

Cover design by Jason Anscomb
Printed in the UK by CMP (UK), Poole, Dorset

Product code – 012025500
This product has been assessed as low risk and can be used safely without safety information.

The manufacturer's authorised representative in the EU for product safety is:
Easy Access System Europe – Mustamäe tee 50, 10621 Tallinn, Estonia
gpsr.requests@easproject.com

Stop F*cking Nodding: and other things 16-year-olds say in therapy

Contents

	Introduction	*1*
1.	Aiming for perfection	*15*
2.	Mud sticks	*36*
3.	Lessons in love	*59*
4.	In transition	*78*
5.	Wanking	*102*
6.	Maturation	*121*
7.	Mother and son	*137*
8.	Learning to live	*154*
9.	Bored and angry (but mostly angry)	*172*
10.	F*cking nodding	*192*
	References	*197*
	Name index	*203*
	Subject index	*205*

About the author

Jeanine Connor is a psychodynamic child and adolescent psychotherapist, clinical supervisor and training facilitator. She has supported young people and those who work with young people in a variety of settings for 25 years. Jeanine is the author of *Reflective Practice in Child and Adolescent Psychotherapy: Listening to young people* (2020), editor of *BACP Children, Young People & Families* journal, reviews editor for the BACP magazine *Therapy Today* and psychology editor for Curriculum Press.

Acknowledgements

I am supremely grateful to every 16-year-old who has spoken to me and to the parents, carers and agencies who support them to do so. Good (enough) therapy owes a lot to good training and supervision, while good (enough) writing owes a lot to good editing. I'm privileged to have had all three.

I would like to acknowledge the wonderful children's charity Place2Be, where my initial training and supervisory support began, following a chance meeting with a discarded copy of *The Times* on the London Underground. My Place2Be tutors set me off on a voyage of discovery: of young people, of the wonderful world of therapy and of myself.

I would like to acknowledge my magnificent tutors at Birkbeck College, who mentored, challenged, critiqued and taught me so much more than the MSc syllabus. They will never know the full influence that they and the course had on me, and I owe them a debt of gratitude. The great psychoanalysts I was obligated to read inspired my early career as a child and adolescent psychotherapist and continue to influence my development now that I choose to read them. They deserve some acknowledgement too.

I would like to acknowledge my clinical supervisor, a candid, critical yet non-judgemental, wise and big-hearted woman who I feel fortunate to learn from and be challenged and supported by.

I should also acknowledge my 16-year-old self, which feels almost as awkward and uncomfortable as she did. She didn't think she was good enough and she still hangs around to remind me of that decades later. Being in supervision, meeting other 16-year-olds every day and writing this book about them have helped me to acknowledge her a little bit more.

Special acknowledgement and appreciation to my editor at PCCS Books, another candid, critical yet non-judgemental woman, who encouraged me to share my stories, reined me in when I needed it and stopped me from becoming clichéd. This book is all the better for her input. Thank you.

Dedication

This book is dedicated, with enormous gratitude, to all the contrary, conflicted, antagonistic, rebellious, divergent, challenging, stroppy, subdued, feisty, bad-tempered, bored, rageful, insightful, inquisitive and amusing 16-year-olds who have allowed me the pleasure and privilege of getting to know them.

Introduction

Sixteen is an interesting place to be. It's where anything can happen and often does; the eye of the storm of adolescence, filled with demands, challenges, turbulence and passion. Sixteen-year-olds are tantalisingly close to adulthood, and to sex and drugs and rock and roll, or at least they think they are, and yet they are still children in the eyes of the law, and will continue to be defined as such, and protected accordingly, until their 18th birthday (OHCHR, 1989). Many 16-year-olds are contrary, conflicted, antagonistic and rebellious. They are often divergent and challenging. Others are sullen and subdued. They are also infinitely interesting, insightful, inquisitive and amusing to those of us who take the time to be interested in and amused by them. I am one of those people.

The book is about some of the 16-year-olds I've met through my work as a child and adolescent psychotherapist. At 16, you are at the epicentre of adolescence, struggling to survive the ordinary upheavals of ordinary teenage life. Peer relationships are intense, and break-ups are devastating. Minor as well as major catastrophes can feel like the end of the world. Many authors, me included, have likened this developmental stage to a stormy sea. The 16-year-olds who arrive in my therapy room are often all at sea.

I have pitched this book at 'the curious and intelligent reader': perhaps a trainee adolescent psychotherapist or counsellor starting out on their career, or a health, education or social care professional working with this infuriating, energising age group, or a parent or carer baffled by the onslaught of unrecognisable thoughts, feelings and behaviours in their own 16-year-old. I have written from a psychodynamic perspective, with explanations of terminology where I feel they might be helpful, but without, I hope, insulting anyone's intelligence. More experienced psychodynamic practitioners will be completely familiar with these concepts, but I want them to be accessible to anyone who knows, loves, is baffled by or is trying to help a 16-year-old in any capacity, and I think the theoretical stuff can help to throw a light on the chaos.

Adolescence is a period of transition, extending from the onset of puberty to about the age of 25. The year we turn from 10 to 11 (usually school year 6) and the year we turn from 15 to 16 (usually school year 11) mark particular periods of transition, from primary to secondary and secondary to tertiary education respectively. These age groups are also under the influence of biology, first through the impact of puberty and, later, through an awareness of sexual potential. This is the ordinary stuff of adolescence and it's a heady mix, tough enough to manage in itself. The more extreme stuff, the stuff that often precipitates psychotherapy referrals, such as self-injury, suicidal ideation, disordered eating and risk-taking behaviour, happens in addition to and in the context of the more ordinary transitional and biological stuff.

Adolescence is also a time when mental health difficulties can come to the fore and are first likely to be diagnosed, with more reported difficulties in females than males and in Year 11s than other year groups (Wright et al., 2020).

The young people I describe in this book are amalgamations of fragments of some of those I have had the privilege to get to know during 25 years in psychotherapeutic practice. I discuss the issues that have fascinated and perplexed me. Of course, it also contains fragments of my own 16-year-old self and her peer group, because all of us carry within us the 16-year-old we once were, and all writing is, at least in part, and not always consciously, autobiographical.

Here I am using the term 'fragment' in its psychological sense. Many of the young people I work with come to psychotherapy feeling unstable, or uncertain about who they are, or confused about what's happened to them. They (and others) might describe themselves as 'broken' or 'damaged' – terms that I'm not keen on because of the negative, passive and permanent connotations. Sixteen-year-olds often present in a state of disintegration. There is an idea that having a self and being a self are states that are stable over time. So, when a young person's sense of self feels unstable, they may have a feeling that they don't know who they are, which can cause them to feel anxious, depressed or suicidal, terrified or overwhelmed. They present as falling or fallen apart, psychologically shattered and often physically exhausted too. These young people's sense of self is unstable because, according to psychodynamic theorists such as Kohut (1971), the structure of the personality has become fragmented. Some of this falling apart fragmentation is an ordinary component of ordinary adolescence. Often, one of my primary tasks as a psychotherapist is to work out with a young person (and their family) how much of what they are experiencing is ordinary developmental stuff and how much of it is something else, so that I can answer the explicit or implicit question, 'Am I going mad?' Sometimes a young person's fragmented state points towards a diagnosable mental illness; often it does not. Either way, normalising and naming what's going on goes a long way towards implementing positive change. So does the experience of the therapeutic relationship, which in and of itself can help a young person to reintegrate those parts of their self that have become fragmented. Early psychodynamic theory emphasised the significance of early childhood and relationships for the successful development of self. However, later theories suggested that development, and therefore integration, continues throughout the lifespan (Elson, 1986), so there is always potential for change and always reason to be hopeful. I truly believe in the potential for change and the power of hope.

In some chapters I've used artistic licence and professional curiosity to imagine parents of clients. In others I've borrowed from narratives about 16-year-olds I've never met in the flesh but have experienced in the transference – the stuff that goes on between a therapist and her client that is unsaid and usually unconscious and that can be informative in helping to understand what's going on in the here and now. Mostly, I've taken a theme of being 16 and embodied it in a 16-year-old from my imagination. Each chapter examines a part of a composite 16-year-old's therapy. There is so much to consider in each and every psychotherapy session – the content (what is said and done), the thinking and feeling (theirs as well as mine), the reflecting, the hypothesising and the formulating, the theoretical considerations and the family context – any one young person's time in therapy could fill an entire book of its own. What I've done here is present a cross-section of 16-year-olds by taking a segment of their therapy, often the bit at the beginning, but sometimes a section from the middle or the end, and putting it under the spotlight, alongside my own psychotherapeutic reflections, to illustrate the ways I try to make sense of what's going on.

Why psychotherapy?

The modality that I trained in and continue to practise is psychodynamic psychotherapy. This doesn't treat the so-called symptoms a young person is struggling with; rather, it aims to make sense of them in the context of their life: past and present, conscious and unconscious. Psychodynamic psychotherapy focuses on each and every aspect of how a young person feels, thinks and behaves, and how I, as their therapist, feel, think and behave in relationship with them. These are the raw ingredients of therapy. My role is to pick out the raw ingredients from the 'soup', examine and explore them, make sense of them, and present them in a way that makes sense to the young person and is easier for them to swallow and digest.

For me, the primary task of therapy is, first and foremost, to listen to what young people have to say. Often, they find it easier to talk to me than they do to their parents (if their parents are around), for a number of reasons: they might think their parents won't or don't understand them, or it might be that they fear reprisal, or they don't want to upset them, so they hold back the full extent of how they're feeling or thinking, or they try to hide what they're up to. Parents or carers are (usually) in a close emotional relationship with their children, and they can't pretend otherwise or switch it off when needs be. That's one of the things young people tell me they find so helpful about a therapist: that they aren't impacted in the same way as a parent or carer by what the young person presents. Not that we aren't affected at all – we wouldn't be very good therapists if we weren't. It's important that we feel something in relation to the young people we work with, and it's equally important, that the young people feel that we feel something.

One of the best bits about offering psychotherapy to young people is getting to know them. But how can I *really* know what it's like to be this particular 16-year-old who is sitting in front of me in this particular room on this particular day, living their own particular version of life? In his paper 'What is it Like to be a Bat?', the philosopher Thomas Nagel wrote that a bat has its own conscious experience, but we cannot imagine what that is like because our imagination is based on our own experience and is therefore limited (Nagel, 1974). This perhaps begs the question of whether it is possible to understand and support a person who has suffered bereavement, or bullying, or depression, or sexual abuse, if the therapist has not experienced that thing themselves.

Can they imagine what something feels like that is beyond their own experience? Nagel argued that the same may be said for other humans as for bats: that there can be the *knowledge* of another person, but he questioned the extent to which there could be an *understanding* of what it is like to have another person's experiences. He argued that his understanding could only go as far as his imagination, which was not very far at all. It could only tell him what it would be like for *him* to be another person, or for *him* to be a bat, not what it was like for another person to be that person, or for a bat to be that bat. I want to know what it is like for this 16-year-old to be this 16-year-old. Is that possible? Is that what we call empathy?

Empathy is the capacity to feel and understand what another person is feeling and understanding from within their own experience and frame of reference. Freud, the founding father of psychodynamic theory and psychoanalysis, only fleetingly mentioned empathy in a footnote in one of his articles: 'A path leads from identification by way of imitation to empathy' (Freud, 1921), which isn't quite the way I see it. Identification can arise in psychotherapy, and when it does, it's important to acknowledge and analyse it, preferably with the support of supervision. As for imitation, I think that would be an obstacle best avoided on the path to understanding and empathy. Psychoanalytic literature had to wait until 1959 for a fuller examination of empathy, in Kohut's paper 'Introspection, Empathy, and Psychoanalysis' (Kohut, 1959). In it, Kohut defined empathy as the ability of one human being to gain access to the psychological states of another human being, and he saw this as the foundation of psychoanalysis. He believed, as do I, that we do have the potential to truly understand what it's like for a person to be that particular person, even if we can't grasp what it's like for a bat to be a bat.

Another important task of psychotherapy is helping to make sense of what often doesn't make much sense at all when I meet a young person and their family for the first time. They, and their worried families and carers, bring questions such as 'Why do I feel like this?', 'Am I mad?', 'Why is he behaving that way?', 'Why has my son tried to end his life?', 'Why is my daughter taking so many risks with her safety?' I start to make sense of things by listening, observing, and being curious; by thinking, linking and reflecting in the here and now as well as in the context of what I learn about the young person's family history and experiences. The young people themselves are the experts about themselves; the family, if they are around, can add valuable context. My understanding of psychological theory and my therapeutic experience provide the wider context that helps me to make sense of what's going on. I name things and I normalise them. I assess and manage risk. I explore the ordinary and the extraordinary thoughts, feelings and behaviours, so that gradually and hopefully I can help the young person make sense of them and put themselves back together again.

In all of this, I am supported by my clinical supervisor, who thinks and reflects with me about the young people I meet, because two heads are usually better than one. Just as psychotherapy is a collaborative process between client and therapist, so supervision is a collaborative process between supervisee and supervisor. All of us need external support to survive the journey. Young people have their parents, or parents *in loci*; therapists have their supervisor, and supervisors have *their* supervisor. Parents sometimes have their own therapist too, or a co-parent or their own parent – everyone needs someone with whom they can be honest about how they're feeling in relation to the task of supporting young people in their particular role.

There's a common adage in therapy that therapists can only take a client as far as they have gone themselves. Some people think that clients can only be helped by therapists who have shared their experience. For example, in order to support a person who has suffered bereavement/bullying/depression/sexual abuse, the therapist must have experienced bereavement/bullying/depression/sexual abuse themselves. I don't think that's what the adage means at all. I think it does (and should) mean that we can only accompany clients on journeys of personal psychotherapeutic exploration if we've travelled that path ourselves. One 16-year-old asked me if I'd had therapy and if so, what for. I told her, 'Yes, I have, because I needed to make sure I had my own shit together in order to be able to help you to get your shit together.' She liked that answer, and said it was good to know that I had 'been in the hot seat' and that I had practised what I preached. I had hoped I wasn't being preachy, but I thought that one over with my supervisor.

How psychotherapy works

So, how do I work with 16-year-olds? The stories in this book illustrate the lived examples, supported by theory. Kazdin defined psychotherapy as 'interventions designed to decrease distress, psychological symptoms and maladaptive behaviour, or to improve adaptive and personal functioning through the use of interpersonal interaction, counselling or activities following a specific treatment plan. Treatment focuses on some facet of how clients feel (affect), think (cognition) and act (behaviour)' (Kazdin, 1990). As definitions go, it's pretty dry, but it sets the parameters.

Psychotherapy is certainly an intervention designed to decrease distress, including distressing psychological symptoms, and it can bring about changes in what are commonly called maladaptive behaviours. I don't offer behaviour modification, although I meet a lot of parents and carers who hope I can stop a young person stealing, or cutting themselves, or engaging in promiscuous sexual activity, or misusing alcohol or illegal substances. The aim of psychotherapy, for me, is to try to help young people to make sense of their behaviour, without condoning or condemning it, without referring to it as maladaptive or bad, and without diagnosing or pathologising it or purposefully trying to stop it. My way of working isn't focused on a solution, although of course I hold any desired hopes and expectations in mind, and these often include an anticipated change in behaviour. Some of the questions I ask during the initial meeting with a young person and their parent or carer are 'Why are you here? Why now? What do you hope to get from therapy? What will that look like? What would change?' I want them to really think about the point of therapy, for them, and how they will know when they are ready to end. Sometimes the expectations differ between parent and child; sometimes they're unrealistic, but that's why it's important to ask the questions and think about the answers before we embark on a therapeutic journey together: we need to know where we're headed so we can recognise when we get there. *My* aim is to bring about an improvement in a young person's capacity to function in a healthier, less risky way. I do this by seeking to make sense of the behaviour and work out why it might be happening.

Cutting yourself, drinking to excess, stealing or having risky sex might appear maladaptive to the adult observer, but I believe that such behaviours must be serving some sort of psychological function for the young person themselves. To put it another way: what might seem self-destructive, even life-threatening, is often what's keeping the young person alive. It's a way they've found to survive, albeit a potentially harmful way, but I respect that.

The 'treatment' part of how I work is the development of the therapeutic relationship, because that's what facilitates change. All the research evidence shows that it's the relationship between therapist and client that matters – not how many sessions they have, or what kind of therapy we practise, or how much training and how many qualifications we've got (Kantrowitz, 2020).

As a psychodynamic psychotherapist, I'm alert to the transference relationship, as well as to the relationship in the room. Transference is what we call the stuff that goes on between two people (not always the therapist and client) that is usually non-verbal and may be left over from past experiences, and can be helpful to consider in relation to what's going on in the here and now. For example, I might find myself having a strong feeling towards a young client in the therapy room – let's say, it's disbelief. They might be telling me about their day, their week or something about their previous experience. It might *sound* all very well and good, all very adolescent, ordinary and plausible, but it might not *feel* quite right, and my thought might be, 'I'm not sure I believe you.' It's important that I notice my thoughts and feelings in relation to the young person I'm working with because these thoughts and feelings may be telling me something about that young person's experience – in this instance, perhaps, their experience of being disbelieved. What emerges in the transference may not necessarily be what they are talking to me about, here and now; it's as likely to be about something else, in a different context, and relate to someone else, in a different relationship.

The transference relationship can be thought of as an 'as if' relationship (Gray, 2014), because the client behaves towards the therapist, particularly at the beginning of the relationship, *as if* they were someone else, often a parent, which creates a counter-response in the therapist *as if* they were the young person's parent. That's transference (or, in this example, parental transference), which is the transfer of feelings from the client about their parent, unconsciously, onto me. Sometimes the transference includes the client's loving or sexual feelings towards someone in the real world. That kind of transference is called erotic transference, and, like parental transference, it can happen in therapy with 16-year-olds too. What I feel in response to the transference is called countertransference: that's a feeling that doesn't belong to me or to the young person, or to the relationship between us in the present, but has nevertheless *got into me*, so that I feel it. When I become aware of a countertransference feeling, the most important thing to do is acknowledge it. I think of these feelings, which are sometimes uncomfortable, as messengers: I need to feel them because they are giving me information about the young person in front of me. Sometimes they make immediate sense, often not, in which case I reflect on them afterwards, or in supervision, or I store them away in my mind for later. There are plenty of examples of how I work with transference throughout this book.

Diagnosis and medication

I'm alarmed by the number of young people I meet who are trailing a string of acronyms attached to their names – ADHD, ODD, ASD, PDA, GAD and BPD,[1] to name a few of the most common – and how many come with a diagnosis of severe mental illness, such as schizophrenia or psychosis. And it's getting more and more common. When I started working with young people in the late 1990s, hardly any of them were diagnosed with anything. Within the space of a generation, the ratio has flipped; now it's the majority who either have or are seeking a diagnosis. And I wonder why.

Some people argue that the rapid escalation in diagnosing young people is due to an increased awareness, a growing understanding, better assessment, more careful observational skills, science. To me, a more convincing argument is that the way we think about young people has changed, as have the social norms, expectations and constructs that define them. As child and adolescent psychiatrist Sami Timimi writes in *A Straight Talking Introduction to Children's Mental Health Problems* (Timimi, 2021), childhood in Western contemporary culture has changed enormously. He cites changes in family structure, lifestyle, the 'domestication' of childhood due to fears about risk (what previous generations might have called 'wrapping kids up in cotton wool'), the use of social media, changes in education, including exams and league tables, and the 'commercialisation' of childhood, parenting and pharmaceuticals. These changes affect our expectations about what normal (and abnormal) childhood looks like, and what is classified as normal (and abnormal) behaviour in young people. Timimi suggests that it is harder than ever to be a 'normal' child.

---

1. ADHD (attention deficit hyperactivity disorder); ASD/ASC (autism spectrum disorder/condition); BPD (borderline personality disorder); GAD (generalised anxiety disorder); ODD (oppositional defiance disorder); PDA (pathological demand avoidance) – all diagnoses that can be found in the *Diagnostic and Statistical Manual of Mental Disorders* (5th edition) (APA, 2013).

If normality is measured by majority, then my fear is that having a mental health diagnosis is fast becoming the norm for children and young people, and that's very worrying.

I find it concerning for two main reasons. First, labels stick. Many young people and their families blindly accept the subjective (in my opinion) and somewhat arbitrary (in my opinion) judgement of the psychiatrist doing the labelling, who often doesn't know them or their family history very well and doesn't have the time or the inclination to get to know them. I think this acceptance of what the psychiatrist says is to do with status. They are a 'proper' doctor and so they must know what they're talking about. Getting a diagnosis can be a relief, and it does have its place, but labelling can also be a lazy way of explaining away what's going on. It is a reductionist approach that (in my opinion) condenses a whole individual into a small set of symptoms.

My second concern is that the increase in the diagnosis of mental illness in children and young people often leads to the use of prescription drugs to treat (or mask) the symptoms (or characteristics) of normal childhood and adolescence, so that ordinary emotional and developmental traits are pathologised and medicated. Of note is a growing body of research that reports very little effectiveness in the prescription medication widely given to children and young people, such as antidepressants, stimulants and antipsychotics (Moncrieff, 2020; Timimi, 2021; Watson, 2019a).

Lucy Johnstone reminds us that the manuals used to diagnose people with mental illness are not supported by robust, scientific evidence and that we are right to question them (Johnstone, 2022). She argues that formulations are far more useful than labels, because they take into account an individual's background and experiences and are based on the client's personal narrative and what it means to the individual to be that individual – considerations that are often obscured by diagnoses. I agree. I too deal in formulations, rather than diagnoses, because they are fluid rather than fixed and they can and do change over time as we learn more about our client and as they change. Gray states that 'psychological understanding is not deductive but observational' (Gray, 2014). I think medical diagnosis is both deductive and reductive. Perhaps one of the reasons diagnoses are mostly favoured by medical professionals is because medics generally don't spend much time with their patients; due to pressure of workload, they will see a patient for a matter of minutes. But formulations are generally favoured by psychotherapists because they take time to develop and because we usually spend an hour a week observing and getting to know a client, over months or sometimes years. I say 'generally' because, as with everything, there are always exceptions.

I'm often asked by clients or parents to diagnose or give an opinion on a diagnosis, but that's not my job. Whether a young person comes with a diagnosis or is seeking one, I approach both scenarios in the same way I do anything else that's 'brought' to therapy. I think about it with the client; I explore it; I open it up it and try to make sense of it with the young person in the context of what is going on, or has gone on, for them in their lives. For example, if someone has a diagnosis of anxiety and has been prescribed anti-anxiety medication, I ask what they understand that to mean, why they've been prescribed the drug and how they think it is helping. Often, they don't understand any of it, because often it hasn't been explained to them. If this is the case, I offer some basic factual information (what professionals might refer to as 'psychoeducation') about diagnosis and how psychiatry works, and about medication and how that is supposed to work. Then I get on with what I'm most interested in, which is what it means to this young person. What does it mean to have been given this diagnosis at this time? Does it make sense to them? How do they feel about taking medication and do they think it's making a positive difference?

I'm worried that psychotherapy, which was originally thought of as a 'talking cure', is becoming more aligned with the medical model of psychiatry, which is mostly interested in what's *wrong* with the person. For me, and many other therapists, what interests us, and is the focus of our work with young people and their families, is *what's happened* to them. The whys and why nots of diagnosis are beyond the remit of this book, but I strongly recommend *Drop the Disorder!* (Watson, 2019b), an edited collection of chapters by professionals and non-professionals challenging the 'psychiatric propaganda' that has led to millions of young people being diagnosed with a 'mental illness' that needs to be 'chemically managed'. One of the contributors, consultant clinical psychologist Lucy Johnstone, asks a question I ask too: 'Do you still need your psychiatric diagnosis?' Lots of young people are nonplussed by this question. Understandably, given the status of psychiatry, they think the label they've been given, the medical definition of their 'illness', has been etched onto them in indelible ink. Or, as one adolescent said to me, 'My BPD goes through me like a stick of rock.' My aim, with that young person and with others, is to try to help them contemplate the idea that a label is just a label and that I'm interested in peeling that label back and exploring with them what's underneath. Sometimes, the response is an angry tirade. I've questioned the identity their diagnosis has given them – the reason for them feeling bad or sad or mixed up or confused; I've questioned if they are 'ill' at all, and who am I to question what they've been told by an actual doctor?

It's important to make these challenges gently because labels can provide certainty and, with it, a sense of safety. We might peek under the corners to explore the histories, hurts and hidden terrors that lie beneath, but we must acknowledge that labels serve an important purpose. I think that sometimes the purpose is avoidance or denial – defences that must be treated with respect, rather than ripped away quickly like a sticking plaster.

Essentially, though, my own experience and a wealth of evidence suggest that diagnostic labels don't make that much difference to the outcome, and nor do the diagnosis or medication. What matters most is that the young person gets to talk to someone who listens to their story. It's the relationship that's the cure.

Why sixteen?

I decided I wanted to focus this, my second book, on 'being 16' when I was researching and writing my first, *Reflective Practice in Child and Adolescent Psychotherapy: Listening to young people* (Connor, 2020). I noticed the referrals I'd received included disproportionately more 16-year-olds, most often girls, and I wondered why. Writing this book is my attempt to answer that question. The developmental stage of adolescence often leaves young people flummoxed and floundering, and the adults around them feeling helpless, not knowing how to respond. As I said at the start of this introduction, adolescence is a period of massive transition, from the perspectives of both nature and nurture. In a period that lasts from the onset of puberty to around the age of 25, 16 is the eye of the storm.

For this book, I decided to embark on an exploration of the challenges faced by 16-year-olds in particular, to share the sense I have made of them and with them, with the aim of helping other people who support 16-year-olds to make sense of them too. I draw on a wide range of literature to develop my thinking and writing, with influences from classic psychoanalytic thinkers, such as Freud (the founding father of psychodynamic theory, who wasn't just obsessed with sex and whose theories are very relevant to understanding the unconscious motivations of young people, even today); Bowlby (the influential attachment theory guru); Klein (who had more to offer than complex object relations theory and ideas about good breasts and bad breasts); Winnicott (hugely influential in regard to the mother/infant relationship), and Bion (the prominent authority in group relations theory). These writers formed the foundation of my training as a child and adolescent psychotherapist. Their ideas and philosophies have shaped the way I think about young people, and they continue to inform my practice. For this book, I also draw from the work of more contemporary psychotherapists and from non-psychoanalytic texts, including feminist writers Susie Orbach and Gloria Steinem, children's author Michael Rosen (*We're Going on a Bear Hunt*) and poet Philip Larkin ('They fuck you up, your mum and dad'), as well as the Urban and Oxford English dictionaries and the latest research in education and mental health. Influences and ideas sometimes come from the strangest of places; sometimes they're really obvious.

The title I've chosen for the book, while deliberately provocative, will resonate with other psychotherapists who work with young people – and probably with many young people themselves, especially those who've been in therapy. These were the words spat angrily at me by Mercedes, a feisty, bad-tempered, bored and rageful 16-year-old who had been sent to me, kicking and screaming, for 'anger management' by her parents and teachers, who were at the end of their tethers. Mercedes turned up, but she didn't want to talk to me; she was too angry, and being sent to therapy made her angrier still. I was told by her pastoral support teacher that Mercedes made everyone's life hell, but that she had a soft spot for her and didn't want to give up on her. I developed a soft spot for Mercedes too, even though she rebuffed all initial attempts I made to get to know her. I asked about school and social life. She told me to fuck off. I asked about home and family. She told me to fuck off. I commented that it seemed like she didn't feel like talking to me much and she told me, 'No fucking shit, Sherlock.'

I decided to hold back on the inquisition and try to show her instead that I totally understood where she was coming from, that I empathised with her reluctance to open up, and that it was okay to talk or not talk. I wanted her to know that I was on her side, that I wouldn't give up on her, and that I was a reasonable, chilled, flexible, amenable, 'here for you' kind of therapist. I did this with the familiar therapist trope: the compassionate, barely-there smile, kind eyes and gentle nods of the head. To which Mercedes demanded, at the top of her voice: 'WILL YOU STOP FUCKING NODDING!' And I knew that I was going to absolutely love working with Mercedes, if she carried on turning up. She did, and I did, but we both came to the realisation early on that individual psychotherapy wasn't right for her. Sometimes it's to do with timing, or match or modality. Sometimes it's something else. My sense was that individual psychotherapy might feel too intimate and intense for Mercedes, and I offered her the opportunity to join a group I'd been asked to facilitate for other 16-year-old girls who were deemed to be 'at risk' – of failing, dropping out and getting into serious trouble of the drugs or alcohol or teenage pregnancy kind. She accepted, and you'll find out how she – and the others – got on in Chapter 9.

If readers recognise their 16-year-old selves or relatives in Mercedes, or any of the other young people I describe in this book, then I've done my job. Most authors tend to include a disclaimer at the start of their book, along the lines of 'individuals and events contained in this work are totally fictitious and any resemblance to actual individuals and events is coincidental'. Quite right too – client work is confidential, and we shouldn't be using it as material. But if we don't share *stories* from our therapy rooms, how will we learn and grow as professionals and how will we be able to pass on our learning to parents and carers and other non-psychotherapists so that they can better understand the adolescents in their care? So, I *do* share stories and experiences, but they are anonymised and unidentifiable.

Equally, I don't believe in coincidence. Of course, we share similar experiences at similar stages in our lives and it can be a great comfort to know this; to know that others have struggled and that they have survived and we can survive too. I hope that readers will identify *parts* of their own clients, or family members, or themselves in these stories, and that they will gain learning, validation and recognition from those identifications. The dialogue is invented (except for 'stop fucking nodding'), as are the names of the individuals and the narratives assigned to them, but the themes are absolutely true.

1

Aiming for perfection

Abebi, Clara, Dot, Fliss and Evie are high achieving, hard-working perfectionists with low self-esteem. Can group work help them to explore the ordinary and not-so-ordinary stuff to do with being 16, and accept that good enough is good enough – as are they?

. . . .

I've already mentioned in my introduction that a disproportionate number of the psychotherapy referrals I receive are for 16-year-olds, and this is why I decided to write this book in the first place. And of those referrals, a disproportionate number are for girls, and many of those girls are affected by low self-esteem. So, 16-year-old girls with low self-esteem make up a large proportion of my caseload at any given time. Like most presenting issues, levels of low self-esteem vary along a continuum, from a mild to moderate sense of not feeling good enough at one end to a crippling feeling of worthlessness at the other. Those at the crippling end of the scale are also likely to display features of anxiety and/or low mood; they may strive for perfection and over-achieve, or they may strive for perfection, fall short and fail. They may withdraw and isolate or act-out, or they may struggle with disordered eating, disordered sleeping, self-injury and thoughts of suicide. In other words, while each of these 16-year-old girls may present differently on the outside, what they have in common on the inside is that they're all feeling like crap.

There are some obvious, ordinary reasons why many 16-year-old girls have low self-esteem. First, most of them, most years – pandemics aside – have exams to contend with. No matter what a young person's academic ability, ambition or potential may be, exams are (usually) conducted in a public sphere, which (usually) feels exposing. There's a lot about exams that's ritualised; again, pandemics permitting, it's been pretty much the same thing, year in, year out, since forever.

Mock exams happen in the winter, the real things take place in the summer. There's a celebration after the last exam, be that a formal prom or an informal bottle of illegally purloined plonk in a park, with the final ritual being the long-anticipated results day towards the end of the long summer break. These exam rituals are linear and predictable, and they are the backdrop to Year 11, the year that these young people turn 16.

In the run-up to the summer exam period, 16- (or almost-16-) year-olds talk about how much or how little revision they are doing, over- or under-exaggerating according to the social norms of their particular peer group. 'Oh, I've hardly done a thing,' says the girl who's hardly done a thing, but the same words are just as likely to be uttered by the girl whose nose has been firmly planted in her books since the beginning of the autumn term. So, no one really knows for sure who's done what or where they fit on the scale of done-enough to not-done-enough. And 16-year-olds do like to know where they fit.

It's not just in terms of exam preparation or results that 16-year-old girls compare themselves with other 16-year-old girls; they compare themselves on everything – clothes, friendships, families, phones, sex, number of followers on social media, number of likes, number of days in their Snapchat streak, number of Snapchat streaks, level of definition achieved in their eyebrows, bra size, dress size, butt size – and those with low self-esteem always decide that they aren't as good as the other girls, even though lots of the other girls are thinking the same about them. This ordinary, everyday stuff is the backdrop to the story I'm going to share with you here.

A particularly astute student support manager from a local secondary school, Miss Martinez, contacted me to discuss her cohort of Year-11 girls. She said she was concerned about their mental health and wondered if they were depressed. They were spending a lot of time in her office, crying, complaining of headaches and stomach aches, and seeming miserable and anxious. Several of the girls were harming themselves and some were talking about suicide. Miss Martinez thought that they seemed lethargic, their weight appeared to fluctuate, and they all had low self-esteem. I doubted that an entire year group of 16-year-old girls could be depressed, but I agreed to meet with Miss Martinez to discuss her concerns, and when I did, I could see her point.

The Royal College of Psychiatrists (RCPsych, 2021) lists some of the symptoms of childhood depression as: being self-critical and self-blaming, becoming withdrawn, moody or irritable, feeling miserable and tearful, eating too little or too much, finding it difficult to concentrate, suffering from aches and pains, feeling you are not good-looking, feeling hopeless and wanting to die. The RCPsych states that, 'if you have all or most of these signs and have had them over a long period of time, it may mean that you are depressed'. It doesn't say how long a 'long period of time' is, and the disclaimer also states that their website provides information rather than advice. The problem I have with this kind of 'information' is that it leads to the pathologising of ordinary adolescent development by well-meaning individuals, which can result in young people being diagnosed with a mental illness and, in some cases, being prescribed antidepressants. My own disclaimer would warn that, rather than being an indication of a childhood mental illness, the RCPsych list covers many of the common 'signs and symptoms' of adolescence *per se*.

I couldn't offer all of Miss Martinez's Year-11 girls individual psychotherapy, and I doubted whether most of them would need it, but we did agree that some of them needed *something* that fell somewhere between student support and psychotherapy. That conversation led to the inception of a small therapeutic group. So Miss Martinez spoke to six of the girls we had identified as suitable for therapeutic support and mooted the idea of group work to them. Five accepted. Once we'd gained the necessary permissions and ironed out the practicalities, I facilitated a six-week group to explore the ordinary and not-so-ordinary stuff to do with being 16 and to try to bolster the girls' waning self-esteem.

Group work

Group work is fascinating. A group is more than the sum of its parts, as anyone who's ever facilitated or participated in one will attest. What happens in individual therapy, as I mentioned in the Introduction, is a complex mix of what the young person brings – their experiences, their relationship with their parents or carers, their relationship with their therapist, including the transference relationship and their thoughts and feelings – as well as the therapist's thoughts and feelings and *their* previous experiences and relationships. Imagine that, multiplied by the number of individuals in a group, who each 'bring' all of their experiences and relationships within and outside of the group.

Within a group, there are various levels of awareness, including what we say we do, what we believe we do but don't always say and what we do unconsciously (Lawrence, 1977). This is a potent mix, and it's important, therefore, to think carefully about who to invite to a group and how it is facilitated. As an analogy, imagine you're planning a big celebration for up to 100 guests. Top of the guest list would undoubtedly be family and close friends, followed by colleagues and neighbours. If you still had space, you might extend invitations to lesser-known acquaintances and friends of friends. You'd be interested in, or at least relaxed about, choosing people of different ages and genders, from different walks of life, with different experiences and different personalities. There'd be so many people at the party that everyone would find someone they either knew already or wanted to get to know. Imagine now that you're planning a more intimate gathering, a dinner party perhaps, for six or eight people. You're more likely to invite like-minded friends, some of whom might know each other and some of whom might not, but who you think will get on. The process of planning the group was more like planning a dinner party than planning a big celebration. I didn't know the girls beforehand, but I'd read the referral forms and I'd chatted to the student support manager, who did know them, and we tried to think about who would fit together (and with me, the host) and how those girls' minds and experiences would interact with each other.

Another important part of the planning was to think about how to present the group and what to call it. Names matter because they say something about identity. I was keen not to call it 'group therapy', which has connotations of illness and treatment. But a group always meets to 'do' something (Bion, 1961) – so, if not treatment, what was it we intended to do? I've run numerous groups and they're always different, so I knew the answer would depend on the particular group of adolescents and that it might be different each time. With this group, in the beginning, I simply called it 'the group', not wanting to project any of my own preconceptions, expectations or meanings onto those who attended. The name 'Girl Gang' came about because this group of girls wanted to give it a name, and it stuck. For this reason, I talk about 'girls', which is in no way intended to infantilise the young women who attended.

Meeting the group

I set out six chairs in a medium-sized office space. I'd initially been offered the school hall or the library: the former was big and felt exposed, with its floor-to-ceiling windows along one side; the latter was cluttered and felt distracting. Getting the space right was important – not too big and not too small; not too bland and not too busy. We needed enough room to sit comfortably in a circle, but not so much space that we would feel on show and un-held. I think the space for individual therapy, supervision or groups should feel warm, comfortable and welcoming, so that the people invited into it feel contained by the space. I accept that it's not always possible to have much say over this, particularly when we are working in shared spaces, as so many of us so often are.

The five girls who'd accepted the invitation to attend all arrived pretty much together at 10am – of course they did, they were compliant young women, bordering on perfectionists. I invited them to come in and take a seat, which they did silently and neatly. What I mean by that is that they put down their things *neatly*, tucking them under their chairs or hanging them on the backs of their chairs, and they positioned themselves *neatly*, choosing a chair without any fuss and sitting upright, as if to attention. My first thoughts about the girls were that they seemed exactly that: neat and compliant. They also looked expectant and somewhat apprehensive. They were used to knowing what was what and how to behave, but this was a new experience. I introduced myself.

'Hello, I'm Jeanine and I'm pleased to see you all here.'

'Hi,' they said, almost in unison (neat) and smiling politely (compliant).

'Perhaps you'd like to introduce yourselves to the group?'

'I'm Fliss.'
'Hello, Fliss.'
'I'm Dot.'
'Hello, Dot.'
'I'm Abebi.'
'Hello, Abebi.'
'I'm Clara.'
'Hello, Clara.'
'I'm Evie.'
'Hello, Evie.'

They'd compliantly and neatly done as I'd asked, no more and no less. These girls needed direction, which is not my usual style. I work in a non-directive way, following the client's lead, but sometimes they need help to get started. I wondered if I could lead the group by modelling rather than commanding – demonstrating what I hoped they would be able to do for themselves. I gave it a go.

'We're meeting together today for our first group, and I'm imagining you have lots of thoughts and feelings about that. I know that I do.' They nodded expectantly but didn't say anything, and so I continued. 'First, I'm feeling pleased that you all turned up!' My attempt at humour was met with polite giggles. 'And I'm also feeling a bit apprehensive.' The girls looked suddenly serious. 'We've never met each other before, we don't know each other, and we don't *really* know what this group is going to be like…'

'I know Evie.' This came from Fliss, and Evie nodded.

Following suit, Clara added, 'I think I've met Abebi before.'

'Yes, I think so too,' Abebi agreed.

'OK, so Evie and Fliss already know each other. Abebi and Clara have met before. What about you, Dot?'

'I don't know anyone.'

A sympathetic 'Ahhh' from the other girls caused Dot to blush.

'You don't know anyone here, Dot?'

She shook her head vigorously, seeming not to want to say anything else, keen not to draw any more attention to herself than my direct question had already provoked.

'Me neither,' I said, feeling a pull to pair up with Dot, who seemed to have been singled out as *the girl who doesn't know anyone*.

'So, perhaps it might be nice, those of you who would like to, to say something about yourself that you'd like the rest of us to know. Anything at all. Your choice.'

My suggestion was met with universal silence.

'Who would like to go first?'

Some of the girls looked around at the others. Dot looked down at her hands. Fliss and Evie started to giggle again, so I encouraged them to say more.

'Fliss and Evie, you've already let us know that you know each other. Can you say more about that?'

Fliss said, 'We have classes together and sometimes we see each other outside of school.'

Evie added, 'Yes, we're friends.'

'You study together, and you're friends,' I clarified.

'Yes', both of them said, in unison, followed by giggles, then an awkward pause.

'I wouldn't say we're friend-friends, though,' Fliss clarified. 'Would you agree, Evie?'

'Oh, yes, absolutely. My main friend is Selma. She's not in this group.' Evie looked around, as if noticing the absence of her friend Selma for the first time.

I asked, 'I wonder what that's like, to not have your main friend here?'

'It's okay. A bit weird, I suppose. We usually do everything together.'

'And for everyone else, does it feel weird to you too, to be here, in this new group, without the people you usually do things with?'

Everyone nodded and voiced their agreement.

'Maybe we could think about that,' I suggested. 'Maybe we could think about why we decided to come here, without our friends, to this weird-feeling group.'

Fliss went first: 'Miss Martinez suggested it.'

'Same for me,' agreed Evie.

'And me,' from Clara.

'Me too,' added Abebi.

'What about you, Dot?' I asked.

'Yes, Miss Martinez.'

'Can any of you say *why* Miss Martinez suggested it, to you five girls in particular?'

Evie said, 'I've been spending more time in her office lately, talking to her about exams and stuff, and she thought it might help. I think that's why.'

This was a brave statement, and the first reference anyone had made to needing support. It seemed important to explore that and ensure that the other girls felt safe enough to contribute. As with individual therapy, I repeated aloud what I'd heard that seemed significant, in a way that invited further responses.

'She thought it might help...?'

'Yes. I've been finding it hard,' Evie said.

'Exams and stuff?' Again, I repeated what had already been shared, both to acknowledge it and to confirm I'd understood.

'Yes.'

I didn't want the metaphorical spotlight to stay on Evie for too long – as with an actual spotlight, that would feel too exposing. So I asked, 'Is anyone else finding exams and stuff hard?'

Everyone said that they were, but they also seemed to physically relax. It was as if, by acknowledging the hard stuff, the group had been given a focus that freed them from the awkwardness of not knowing what to do or say, so they could *get on with something*. What was beginning to take shape, in those initial, awkward interactions, was the purpose of the group.

'Maybe having a space to think about the hard stuff together each week will be helpful,' I suggested. 'And maybe things will start to feel less hard?'

The girls nodded in unison, neatly and compliantly.

Before we ended our first session together, I thought with the group about our boundaries – things like the time and place of the meeting, the number of sessions planned and the rules around confidentiality, just as I would with a client in individual therapy.

Group task

Wilfred Bion, psychoanalyst and writer, greatly influenced our thinking about group processes. His work with traumatised soldiers during World War II and his role in officer selection helped to form the basis of his theories, which were published in a collection of papers titled *Experiences in Groups* (Bion, 1961). It is true that 16-year-old girls have little in common with soldiers who've served on the front line, but Bion's ideas can still inform the way we think about what goes on in all kinds of groups, and they informed the way I thought about this one. When a group meets, it does so for a specific task, what Bion called the 'working group', which denotes the unconscious fantasy the group has about its purpose.

My fantasy was that the group could provide a holding environment for the girls, as well as a space for reflection and creative exploration. I wanted the group to provide a good-enough container to support the individual identities of its members, while providing them with resources to endure whatever difficulties might arise. But I was aware that a group also has the potential to become an 'arena for crisis' and that it can disintegrate and fall apart (Van Buskirk & McGrath, 1999). My fear was that the girls' individual worries and anxieties would become contagious and that the group experience might do them more harm than good. Every group has an impulse to work and collaborate effectively. But it also has an impulse *against* work, based on the desire to be protected from anxiety (Roberts, 1994).

One of my tasks, as group facilitator, was to try to ensure that the group's impulse to work, collaborate, support and resource its members was balanced with its potential to provoke anxiety, become chaotic and fall apart. I wanted to be able to fulfil this balancing act without being too directive. This task and this dilemma were not so different to those I face in individual psychotherapy, and, as with individual therapy, they were shared responsibilities that often felt like individual burdens. The 'tasks' of therapy and of group work are always shared; I *know* that, but if the group was unsuccessful, whatever that might mean, I knew it would *feel* as if it was my fault, and I was keenly aware of this feeling from the very start. The worst-case scenario was that the girls would gain nothing from the experience (or even feel worse), and the school would withdraw consent and refuse to fund more therapeutic groups in the future.

I think some of what was going on here was about my desire to get it right for the girls, but because my fear of getting it wrong was so powerful, I thought there might also be a parallel process happening that was to do with the girls' projections. What I mean by that is, it was as if something of *their* anxiety about getting it right, and *their* desire to succeed, and *their* fear of failure had got into me. One of the primary tasks of groups (and of therapy) is to hold and make sense of what is going on for the group members (or the individual client) until they are able to hold and make sense of it for themselves. If we are good enough facilitators (or therapists), we do this by using our own thoughts and feelings as a container for the projections (Bion, 1962). I use the term 'good enough' intentionally, as a reminder that good enough is good enough, even though that's sometimes difficult to believe, for the girls in the group, as well as for me, and perhaps for you, too.

Group process

It has been suggested that the psychodynamic method of observing groups involves paying attention to three aspects: objective events, emotional atmosphere and countertransference (Hinshelwood & Skogstad, 2000). Objective events are the group content, the things that happen in reality, in the room. Emotional atmosphere relates to the feelings in the room that belong to the group members, which are less tangible and more subjective. Countertransference is a feeling I feel that doesn't belong to me or the young people in the here and now, but is a response to the transfer of feelings from the group onto me. As I said in the introduction, I find it helpful to think of the transference relationship as an 'as if' relationship (Gray, 2014), because the group behaves towards me 'as if' I was someone from outside the group, which creates a feeling in me 'as if' I was that someone.

What I'd observed already, from the very start of our first meeting as a group, was the emergence of several pairings. Fliss announced that she knew Evie, and Evie confirmed it – pair one. Clara and Abebi said they'd met before, forming a second pair. And when Dot said she didn't know anyone, I said I didn't know anyone either, forming a pair with her. Psychodynamic analytic theory suggests that 'pairing' is the basic assumption most prevalent in therapy professions (Stokes, 1994), as evidenced in this series of brief interactions. So, rather than six individuals, we quickly became a group of three pairs, which, symbolically, has a very different purpose. Bion (1961) suggests that when a 'couple' forms within a group, it is for the purpose of reproduction or creation. He also suggests that the other group members usually behave as if they share the assumption that the primary couple is engaged in intercourse, ignore them, as they would ignore the 'primal scene', and become impotent. He is talking symbolically, but it is interesting to note that what happened in this group was the opposite of this basic assumption. Once the first pair was established (Fliss and Evie), another pair was immediately formed (Clara and Abebi), and then another (Dot and me), perhaps as a challenge to the symbolic status of the primary, and therefore most potent and powerful, couple. I knew that these girls were aspirational and ambitious high-achievers with a desire to do their best and be the best – if I'm honest, I know that about myself, too – and so it makes sense that they/we would challenge, albeit politely and subtly, any competition that threatened their/our position in the top spot. I had a new theme to be aware of – rivalry.

If I think back even further, the very first pair was formed when I'd wondered about why the girls had come, and Fliss mentioned Miss Martinez, a member of staff, and therefore, perhaps, a more powerful partner for her to form a pair with than any of the other girls would be. I also noticed that Fliss had usually been the first person to respond to any comment or question from me – perhaps that was an attempt to form a powerful pairing too, by claiming me as her partner. Alternatively, I wondered if she was trying to establish herself as group leader, and how the others would respond to that. Soon after Fliss initiated the pairing with Evie, she separated herself from it – 'I wouldn't say we're friend-friends, though' – perhaps communicating that there was only room for one girl at the top.

The one time that Fliss hadn't been the first to comment was when I wondered about why Miss Martinez had suggested the group to each of the girls. It was Evie who'd said she'd been 'spending more time in her office', perhaps in an attempt to usurp Fliss (unconsciously) in the primary pairing. But she'd also admitted, courageously, that she'd been there to talk about 'exams and stuff' that she'd been finding hard, illustrating her vulnerability and demonstrating that she was less of a threatening rival.

Girl Gang

When we next met, the girls again arrived on time and sat in the same seats in the same neat way as in week one. I acknowledged that it was our second meeting, that we'd learned each other's names and why we had come, and I wondered aloud how they'd like to use the space.

Fliss announced, 'We need a name!'

'A name?' I wondered.

'Yes. *We* all have names, obviously, but the group doesn't have one. We should give the group a name.'

I asked what everyone else thought about Fliss's idea and the girls agreed it was a good one.

The task of thinking about the group name took up most of the session. While I acknowledge the potential significance of this, in terms of identity and a desire to belong, at the time I also wondered if it was an attempt to defend against anxiety and an illustration of the impulse *against* the primary task of the group, which had been acknowledged as having a space to think about the hard stuff. Maybe the hard stuff was too hard to think about just yet and thinking of a name was a way of delaying it. After a considerable amount of verbal to-ing and fro-ing, and a substantial amount of colourful lettering on the whiteboard, the girls settled on *Girl Gang* – a name they unanimously declared to be 'perfect'.

I was curious, as I always am, about the semantics: the choices of 'girl' and 'gang'. Theoretically speaking, there is a difference in meaning between a gang and a group. Gangs require uniformity; they say, 'We are the same and if you're not in our gang, you're different to us; you're the enemy'. An important function of a gang, by extension, is to protect its members from feeling vulnerable and dependent (Kegerreis, 2010). The choice of 'girl' seemed contradictory. It can be perceived as infantilising and has connotations of the very vulnerability and dependence that 'gang' could be attempting to disavow. It was also, perhaps, a communication that these young women, on the verge of adulthood, were exerting their right to say when (and how) they would transition from girl to woman. They were more than the sum of their hormones. On reflection, I think the paradoxical nature of the name, the joining up of vulnerability, dependence and physical immaturity (girl) and the defence against vulnerability and dependence (gang) *was* perfect, because it encapsulated the essence of mid-adolescence and that inbetweenness, between childhood and adulthood. The name also reminded me of the potential of all groups to become gangs, and to fluctuate between gang and group functioning (Canham, 2002).

Losing their minds

When we met for the third time, there was something about the group that felt different, which I was aware of almost straight away. I greeted the girls as they arrived and took their places. Fliss was slightly early and slightly flustered, said she needed the loo and left the room. Abebi came in and hung her bag carelessly on the back of the chair, and when it fell on the floor, she left it there. Clara placed her water bottle beside her feet, kicked it over, and left it lying on its side. Dot, who I hadn't particularly noticed coming in, seemed to sink down inside her coat, which she had zipped up to her nose, so that only her watchful eyes were peeping out over the collar. Evie was a few minutes late, and came in with Fliss when she returned from the bathroom. None of these things might seem important to the casual observer – a minute here or there, an untidy bag, a horizontal water bottle. But to me, observing from a psychodynamic perspective, both the objective events and the changed emotional atmosphere were significant (Hinshelwood & Skogstad, 2000). Things weren't as neat in the room as they usually were, which suggested to me that things weren't as neat in the girls' internal and external worlds either.

'How is everyone today?' I asked tentatively.

Evie seemed to answer for everyone when she replied, 'Stressed,' and the other girls nodded.

'Stressed how?' I asked

'Stressed to the max,' Abebi clarified. 'We just found out we're doing practice mock exams in *three weeks*!'

'Oh.' I didn't know what else to say.

'I know, right?' It seemed enough. Or at least my facial expression of confusion was enough for Fliss to think I'd picked up on *their* confusion.

'And they only just told us,' Clara clarified.

'I wonder why?' I wondered aloud.

'We don't know, but it's so unfair.'

'I can't bear it,' Dot whimpered, barely holding back her tears. 'I'm losing my mind.'

'This is really affecting all of you,' I said, stating the obvious.

They all nodded, and then spent much of the session expressing their sense of unfairness, the lack of time they had to prepare, their feelings of being set up and their ultimate fear of failing.

I noticed the use of 'they' to denote the nameless bearer of bad news, while the girls used 'we' rather than 'I' to share their thoughts and feelings, as if they had homogenised into one being, united against the common 'they' enemy. Dot had made a painful remark – 'I'm losing my mind' – owning it for herself, but it felt to me as if this was true for all the girls, who seemed now to have one group mind rather than five individual minds of their own. Psychodynamic theory suggests that, when there is anxiety in a group, the group functions in fight/flight mode (Roberts, 1994), in much the same way that an individual might function in a situation where there is perceived threat. The threat I'm talking about here is psychological rather than physical, of course, but the mind, or the group mind in this case, doesn't distinguish. A threat had been identified by the girls, raising their anxiety and igniting their defences to fight it or try to escape. In the opening part of the session, there was tension between these two positions. Dot illustrated her desire to flee (into her coat) and disappear. Fliss fled the room (to go to the bathroom) and Evie was late (had already fled). But then the group became unified in (or by) their shared sense of unfairness and united in their 'fight' against the enemy.

I thought about the chaos and confusion I'd witnessed: the coming and going, the lateness, the carelessness and untidiness. This was a big deal for this particular group of girls, who were known for their compliance, neatness and perfection. In this particular session, they seemed to fall apart. It was as if the primary task of the group had been redefined as providing a container for chaos and confusion, as well as anxiety. Groups function as a whole in relation to other wholes (Bion, 1961), so this was achieved by locating the 'badness' outside of the group in the whole school system, in order to preserve the whole group as a 'good' and safe place (Roberts, 1994). I think it's interesting to note that the group was physically located inside the school setting, because the use of fight/flight functioning can also serve to establish a boundary around a group, separating us from them, good from bad, group from school, cocooning the girls in a safe space. Once I was aware of the origin of the girls' anxiety (the announcement of practice mock exams), the chaos made sense. They were using the safe space created by the group to demonstrate their imperfections and to split off the 'bad' from themselves, illustrating their biggest fear of all – that they wouldn't be good enough.

When someone is missing

The next week the girls arrived punctually and politely, perfection reinstated. Except for Dot, who was missing. As always, there was both a literal explanation – Dot's absence from school – and a theoretical one. Thinking about Dot's absence symbolically, it was as if she had either succumbed to the desire to flee, or she had been expelled. I'd observed her from the start as a quieter, more solitary member of the group, and in the previous session she had told us she was losing her mind, while evidently attempting to disappear into her coat. According to Bion, anxiety in groups can lead to a 'double danger' of either being swallowed up and losing oneself – Dot's experience in the preceding session – or being isolated and removed – symbolised by Dot's absence the following week. So, while I knew that Dot's absence from school probably had a straightforward explanation, symbolically it was significant and worth exploring. After the usual settling in and salutations, I named this for the group.

'No Dot today…'

Clara said, 'I think she's sick.'

'I'm sorry to hear that,' I replied, and then asked, 'I wonder how it will feel to not have her with us today?'

'It's weird, there's always been five of us – well, six if we count you.'

Fliss had attempted to split me off, unconsciously aligning me with Dot so that perhaps I too could be removed from the group.

Although I knew that the girls were all 16, Dot seemed younger to me. She was smaller and quieter and took up less space, physically and verbally, than the other girls did. In this session, because she was absent, she took up no space at all, but, as is the way in experiential groups of this sort, we left her chair in the circle to acknowledge that she had a place here, and her absence seemed to have more of an impact than her presence had.

Abebi said, 'I like Dot.'

'Me too, Clara agreed, 'She's sweet.'

'Sweet?' I wondered.

'Yes, she seems, I'm not sure, like a really sweet girl. Do you know what I mean?'

'Yes.' Evie knew what Clara meant, and agreed, 'She's really sweet.'

'She doesn't say much though,' Fliss stated, seemingly rattled by the praise and the sweetness that was being heaped onto Dot.

'No, but when she does, she seems really honest, you know? Really brave.' Evie was making a stand.

'Brave?' wondered Fliss. 'How is she brave?'

'Like last week when she cried and said she was losing her mind. That was brave.' Evie seemed to be challenging Fliss now.

'I suppose,' Fliss conceded, but then changed her mind. 'But you could say that was weak.'

'Weak?' Abebi was incredulous. 'How is it weak so say how you feel? Isn't that why we're here?' She looked to me to answer the question.

'Is that why we're here?' I repeated to the group, 'To say how we feel?' No one looked certain and there was a contemplative silence as they mulled the question over, before Abebi continued, 'But if someone says they're losing their mind, who are we to decide if that's brave or weak?'

Clara said that was a good point, while Evie nodded her agreement.

Fliss wasn't letting go, though. 'Well I think it's weak. I think once you've lost your mind, you've lost everything!'

'Wow,' I said, 'That's a bold statement, Fliss. Can you help us to understand what you mean by that?'

'Well, our mind is what makes us. So, if we lose it, we lose ourself, we lose who we are, you know.'

'I see what you mean.' I did. 'What does everyone else think? Is it our mind that makes us *us*?'

This led to one of those discussions I love having with 16-year-olds – discussions that fall somewhere between philosophy and existentialism, with a sprinkling of teenage angst. The girls took us round and round and off at random tangents with familiar rhetorical questions such as 'How did we get here?' and 'Are we all made of stardust?', which eventually led to a statement from Abebi: 'So if we're just these miniscule dots floating around on an enormous planet that we're destroying with our consumption of *stuff*, why the hell are we losing our shit over *mock* mock exams?' It was a good point. The girls had found their minds again, and their capacity to think and prioritise and put things into perspective. This had been a collaborative process, but they had used their own individual minds rather than what I'd thought of the previous week as the collective group mind.

Bion didn't perceive such a thing as a group mind, but he believed that, when a group seems to be functioning in such a way, it is a symptom of regression (Bion, 1961). Had the girls regressed the previous week? Had they been infantilised by the threat of exams and retreated into an earlier stage of childhood in order to delay the inevitable? Had they grown up this week, and caught up with their 16-year-old minds?

As I tidied away the chairs after they'd left, I reflected on the session and remembered Dot's absence. I realised that, after the initial acknowledgement, she hadn't been mentioned again, and I found myself feeling guilty that she'd been pushed out, or that the group had colluded with her absence in some way. If this were the case, unconsciously of course, there must be a reason; Dot not being there must have served a purpose. I wondered how the session would have been different if Dot *had* been there and whether and how she would have joined in. I'd begun to think of her as the baby of the group, maybe even the 'cry baby' because she was the only one who had shed any tears. Thinking about process, I wondered if the group needed baby Dot out of the way in order for them to be grown up and have the grown-up discussions they'd needed to have.

The group family/the family group

The following week, our penultimate session, the girls arrived looking relaxed and chatted comfortably to each other as they took their seats.

'Hi girls. Welcome back, Dot.' I said, in greeting.

'Hi. Sorry about last week,' Dot replied.

'There's no need to apologise,' I assured her, then checked, 'Is everything okay?'

'Sort of.'

'Is there anything you'd like to us to know about?' I asked, aware that all eyes were on her.

'I had to look after my brother because my mum was unwell.'

'I'm sorry to hear that,' I said, 'I hope she's better soon.'

'She'll never be better. She's got ME. Sometimes she just has to sleep, and my brother wasn't at school, so I had to stay home to watch him because he's only six.'

Dot had shared more in that statement than she had in all the group sessions to date: that she had a physically unwell mother, that she had care commitments at home and that, seemingly, there was no one else, no father, to share the responsibility. I was reminded of a phrase (which I'm tentatively assigning to Bion), 'a hermit can only be understood in relation to the group from which he separated'. I wondered if the way to better understand Dot (the hermit), to understand all the young women in the group, and, indeed, all adolescents who are in the process of separation, was in relation to their family group.

When I work with individual young people in therapy, I always meet them first with a parent or carer and ask about their family, or family of origin, and their experiences within that family. This sets up the context for what's happening in the here and now. As the psychoanalyst Donald Winnicott wrote, 'Home is where we start from' (Winnicott, 1986a). When I work with groups, I don't meet the parents or include the family in the therapeutic process – at least, not in reality – but the family is always present, in some way, in the group process. Because Dot had 'brought' her family to the session explicitly, I decided to take up the theme explicitly too.

'Thank you for sharing that with us, Dot, so that we have a better understanding about why you weren't here last week.' Then I asked the group, 'I wonder if what Dot has shared has brought up any thoughts for anyone else?'

'It sounds like you've got it hard,' Evie commented. 'I can't imagine what that's like for you, having so much responsibility.'

Dot didn't respond.

'What about your dad? Why can't he look after your brother?' Fliss asked, rather bluntly, what I'd been wondering myself.

'My dad doesn't live with us,' Dot answered.

'Neither does mine,' Fliss replied gently, offering Dot a tender smile of camaraderie.

Abebi asked, 'Do either of you see your dads?'

'I don't,' Dot replied matter-of-factly.

Fliss said, 'I do sometimes, but he's a bit shit.'

'A bit shit how?' I wondered.

'A bit shit in that he doesn't always show up when he's meant to. A bit shit in that he forgot my birthday. A bit shit in that he doesn't give my mum any money for us.'

'Us?'

'My brother and me.'

'Yes, that does sound a bit shit,' I agreed. 'So, we have one shit dad and one unseen dad.' I clarified what Fliss and Dot had shared, using their language, and waited for one of the other girls to contribute.

'My dad's lovely.' Evie seemed almost apologetic.

'That's great,' I reassured her. 'Lovely how?'

'He's kind, supportive, easy to talk to. I talk to him more than my mum, really.'

'My dad's nice too,' Clara added, 'but there's some stuff I wouldn't talk to him about that I tell my mum.'

'Such as?' I wondered.

'Girly stuff, you know, stuff with my friends or if I like a boy.'

'Oh god, I could *never* tell my dad if I liked a boy!' Abebi exclaimed, 'He'd go insane!'

'Insane?' I wondered.

'Literally insane. He'd go mental. There was this boy who my older sister liked, and he liked her. I think they were seeing each other, sort of. Anyway, my dad found out they were talking to each other and he went MAD.'

'What's that about?' Fliss wanted to know.

'He started yelling and shouting, "No daughter of mine is going to behave like a whore while she's living under my roof".' Abebi did an exaggerated Nigerian male accent. 'He took her phone, and her TV and wouldn't let her out of the house for months. It was crazy.'

'What was that like for you?' I asked.

'Well, it taught me what to do when I started talking to boys.'

'Which was?'
'Make sure my dad doesn't find out!'
The other girls sniggered, but I realised that Abebi was serious.
'So how do you talk to boys without your dad finding out?' Clara wanted to know.
'I delete my chat history, like, every five minutes.'
'I do that too,' Clara said. 'I think my parents check my phone. There's nothing bad on there or anything but...' she trailed off and I decided to fill the gap.
'But there's some things that are private.'
'Absolutely,' Clara agreed.

The group shared stories of house rules, family interventions, privacy and lack of it, responsibility and lack of it, siblings and lack of them. As I began to learn about the family constellations of the five girls I'd started to know, I could see how they'd been shaped by them. The family is the first group we belong to and the ways we behave in groups and cope with them, or not, have their roots in family experiences (Kegerreis, 2010). I was interested in how the girls' experiences in their actual families might relate to the positions they'd taken up and the ways they related in the 'group family', and what we could learn about one from the other.

Dot had caring responsibilities for her mother and brother. With one parent absent and the other physically disabled, she'd had to step up and become a sort of parental figure to her sibling and a substitute partner to her mother. In the group, she was able to step down, to relinquish those responsibilities and become the 'baby'. At home, she had to be 'present' to make up for the absences – of a dad and of a healthy mother – but in the group, she had allowed herself to disappear into the background, let others take the lead and even, on one occasion, be literally absent. I could see that how she chose to behave in the group was a way to take a break from the way that circumstances dictated she had to behave at home.

Fliss lived with her mum, who was 'okay', while her older brother was at university and her dad lived somewhere else and was 'a bit shit'. In the initial group session, she had been the first person to form a pair. At home, she was in a pairing with her mother. In the group, she had quickly rejected a pairing with (sibling) Evie, like her own sibling had 'rejected' her when he left home. Fliss had tried instead to form a pair with Miss Martinez or me, recreating a pairing with an adult female that was familiar to her. It was her idea to name the group, suggesting that identity really mattered to her. I wondered if there was a link between this need to identify the group and join its members together with a 'family' name and the absence of her dad and her brother.

Abebi had five siblings: a younger sister and an older sister, who lived at home with her and their parents, and three older brothers, who had left home. In the group, she didn't usually take the lead but she often took a central role in the discussion and had raised some interesting and powerful points: asking whether showing your emotions was brave or weak, and whether, if we're just miniscule dots floating around an enormous planet, why we would lose our shit over exams. In the family, she was the middle girl. In the group, she had taken up the familiar position of the middle girl too.

Evie was an only child who got on well with both her parents but had always longed for a sibling. She was the person to name the struggle with 'exams and stuff' in session one, leading the way for the others to admit their own struggles. She came across as kind and nurturing, describing Dot as 'sweet' and 'honest' and 'brave' – she had the qualities of a lovely big sister, perhaps modelled on her 'lovely' dad.

Clara had a sister who was two years older than her, and they lived with their 'normal mum and dad'. I reflected that, in the group, her contributions often supported whatever the primary speaker said, as if she was following the lead of a 'big sister', most often Abebi. When Abebi said she liked Dot, Clara agreed that she liked her too. When Abebi raised the idea about bravery or weakness, Clara said it was a good point. When Abebi said she deleted her chat history, Clara said she did too. Unintentionally, Clara had placed herself in the role of little sister to big sister Abebi.

The child or young person is always part of a family (Winnicott, 1986a) and the family is always part of them. We carry the family in our minds and behave in ways that both repeat familiar patterns and attempt to make up for actual or perceived losses in acts of reparation. This is true in all aspects of our lives but is perhaps most striking when we come together in groups.

The group is where we start from

Our final group session had been scheduled for the Monday of the week that would now involve practice mock exams. I wondered (and worried about) how the girls would be feeling and whether they would even turn up. They did turn up, and they said they were feeling surprisingly okay. Their anxiety had been tamed and they no longer needed to fight or flee from 'the enemy', as embodied by the school system and the exam system, or some other system that was 'them', not 'us'. They had worked things out and found a clearer perspective. They understood that exams were important; mock exams, slightly less so; mock-mock exams, less important still. They felt less overwhelmed, more able to manage and ready to do their best, knowing and feeling that their best would be good enough.

Girl Gang was born out of a conversation with a student support manager who was worried that her Year 11s were presenting with low levels of self-esteem and symptoms of depression. A group of five 16-year-olds (plus me) met together in the same room at the same time for one hour a week for six weeks. There were very few rules. There was absolutely no agenda. The only expectations were self-imposed and fluid, rather than externally determined and fixed. The girls could choose to attend or not. They could contribute verbally or in silence. They could bring whatever they chose to bring or nothing at all. The girls presented as neat, polite and compliant. We talked about 'the hard stuff' and they allowed themselves to 'lose their minds' and fall apart. The group provided a holding environment and a space for reflection and creative exploration. It allowed the girls to acknowledge and work through their anxiety, rediscover their minds and play with concepts of vulnerability and (in)dependence. My primary task, as group facilitator, was to use *my* mind as a container, to hold the girls and try to make sense of what was going on for them and between them, by paying attention to both the objective events and emotional atmosphere in the room, as well as my countertransference.

The girls didn't feel so alone, so rivalrous, or so inferior. They weren't depressed; they were ordinary, adolescent girls managing ordinary adolescent angst. The experience of being part of a group where they could play out, work through and make sense of their fears and fantasies in a safe, facilitated space had been all the therapy they'd needed. It was perfect.

2

Mud sticks

Kenzie has been accused of sexual assault. Again. His mum describes him as a little shit, and he seems to have been set up to repeat family history. Can therapy help him to contemplate a future that's different to the past?

. . . .

Kenzie's mother, Maria, emailed me. She told me that she needed advice about 'how to control' her 16-year-old son, and that he needed professional help to 'sort himself out'. This type of language isn't unusual at the time of referral; parents and carers are often at their wits' end by this point, although I admit that my hackles rose a bit and my heart sank slightly. It's not in my remit to 'sort someone out' or advise how they can be controlled, and so I emailed back to Maria saying, 'Thank you for contacting me. I'm sorry to hear that your son is struggling. I'd be grateful if you could complete the attached referral form so that I can learn some more about the current situation in the context of your family's history, and then, if you would like, I can offer an initial consultation for the three of us to meet together and explore things some more.'

She replied, 'I'd rather not fill in your form. Can't we just meet? And as soon as possible? He's out of control.'

I found Maria's response a bit abrupt and wondered about her reluctance to complete the referral form. In it, I request basic demographic information, such as address, date of birth and school details, as well as an outline of the referrer's concerns and significant experiences and interventions. I also ask about their hopes and expectations for therapy and how they will recognise if and when they have been achieved. The answers to these last two questions are particularly informative and are elaborated on through discussion at the initial consultation. My intention is to help the referrer to be realistic in their expectations of psychotherapy. I don't have a magic wand and I can't prescribe a magic pill. I'm asking the referrer, often a parent or carer, to think about why they are asking for therapy for the young person from me, right now; what they hope they will get out of it and what that will look like if it works. I was trying to ask Maria what 'sort himself out' actually meant for Kenzie.

If, after I've met with a family for the first time, we decide to work together, the information about hopes and expectations will form the basis of regular therapy reviews, giving us something tangible to refer back to. Something like, 'I remember you said you wanted X to spend more time with the family and less time getting into trouble with his peers. I'm wondering how that's been going since we last met?' Or, 'In the referral, you were hoping that Y wouldn't be so emotionally up and down and that they would be sleeping better. Can you tell me if there have been any changes in their mood or sleep patterns over the last few weeks?' These questions allow me to make qualitative assessments about whether therapy is working for the young person, or not. It's important to note that sometimes a sign that therapy is working is that things look like they're getting worse before they look like they're getting better. This is because therapy can stir up thoughts, feelings and memories that a young person has been trying not to think, feel or remember, and these can manifest in their behaviour. It can also stir up thoughts, feelings and memories for the parent of a young person in therapy too.

Some therapists use quantitative assessments to measure progress and outcomes. They'll ask their clients to complete, or complete with them, strengths and difficulties questionnaires (SDQs), and other such formal measures for anxiety (GAD-7) or depression (PHQ-9). These routine outcome measures (ROMs) can be useful, as they provide a numerical score at the point of referral – a starting point, if you like – and a comparison score at different points along the therapeutic timeline and at the end. Numbers are easy to compare; some people think that whether the number has gone up or down can tell us whether what's happened in therapy has made things better or worse and by how much. Organisations such as school counselling and child and adolescent mental health services (CAMHS) tend to use ROMs, as do GPs and inpatient hospitals. They provide a quick and easy way of producing data about clinical need and therapeutic outcomes that can be used to plan treatment and commission services.

The problem with ROMs is that they don't take into consideration the nuances of the individual's needs and the nature of their lived experiences. They are also biased. Self-report questionnaires may be completed honestly, or they may be a complete fabrication. What if a young person who has been asked to fill in a strengths and difficulties questionnaire doesn't want to engage with services? Easy – they just tick the boxes in a way that demonstrates they have no difficulties and don't need any formal support. What if, on the other hand, a young person really wants one-to-one therapy but has been told they don't need it or they don't meet the criteria? Simple – they just up the ante on the depression questionnaire, to 'prove' that they do. I've seen this happen. I once gave an SDQ to a young man who had been sent a screening form for anxiety. He looked up the diagnostic criteria online and copied it onto the screening questionnaire, so that he effectively ticked every single box for an anxiety disorder. Another young person scrawled all over the questionnaire, 'None of your fucking business'. I'll let you work out for yourself what they thought about therapy.

As I work in private practice, I can hone my referral form and regularly review it, so that it is, and remains, a useful, valuable, workable tool. It's not fail-safe, which is why I meet with the young person and their parent or carer for an initial consultation, to discuss the form and elaborate on the content, but it's a good starting point.

I wondered why Maria was unwilling and/or unable to share any information with me before meeting and what that might mean for ongoing psychotherapy if I were to work with her son. I considered some possibilities: did she have difficulty filling in forms, perhaps practically or psychologically? Was she worried about confidentiality? Or was she intentionally withholding information from me? As is quite common in therapy, I was left in a position of not knowing, holding these unanswered questions until we could meet.

Withholding

After considerable to-ing and fro-ing – it seemed that Maria and I had different understandings of 'as soon as possible' as she rejected several appointments offered and didn't respond to others until the dates had passed – we set up an initial consultation. In my mind, this appointment was, as I'd suggested, 'for the three of us to meet and explore things some more'. Maria's idea of the appointment was different. At the designated time on the designated day, I opened the door to find a slightly built, middle-aged, white woman standing alone on the threshold.

'Maria?'

'Yes. Are you Jeanine?'

'Yes, please come in.'

Once we were inside and seated, I stated the obvious: 'No Kenzie.' Maria stated the obvious too: 'No, I didn't bring him. I thought it was best to come on my own so I can speak honestly about him.'

Up went my hackles and down went my heart again. Maria thought it best not to bring her son to his own initial therapy consultation – what was *that* about? First, she had withheld information and now she was *literally* withholding her son!

'That's interesting,' I said, 'I'm wondering how Kenzie feels about you coming here without him...'

'He doesn't know I'm here. I didn't tell him.'

'You didn't tell him about this appointment?'

'No.'

'What about that you'd contacted me, does he know that?'

'He knows I've been trying to find someone to sort him out, but I didn't tell him I'd found *you*. I wanted to meet you first to see what you were like.'

She was right to want to suss me out; the match between therapist and client is a significant factor in the success of therapy. But so is honesty. Still, I decided it wasn't the time to fight that particular battle. The truth was, I didn't want to get into any kind of battle with Maria, and so I tried to get on with the task at hand.

'Can you tell me why you decided to contact me about Kenzie?'

'He's been accused of rape. Well, sexual assault. He's a little shit, don't get me wrong, but he wouldn't do that.'

'He's been accused of sexual assault. That sounds awful.'

'Yeah. And it's not the first time, either. I've told him, mud sticks, and he's gonna end up locked up at this rate.'

Although I was both alarmed and intrigued, it's not my job to investigate or pass judgement. I was concerned for Kenzie (as well as for his alleged accusers, of course), but if I was going to offer him therapeutic support, I needed to establish first and foremost that it would be ethically and legally appropriate to do so. Concern has been expressed that therapy, and interpretative psychotherapy in particular, can present evidential problems in ongoing crime investigations. The worry is that the outcome of a criminal trial could be tainted if witnesses, and in particular child witnesses, have explored the details of an alleged crime in therapy (Crown Prosecution Service, 2020). Occasionally, I find out about an ongoing investigation during the course of long-term psychotherapy, which poses an ethical dilemma about whether or not to continue. There is less of a dilemma if I'm told about an investigation before commencing therapy, as was the case in this instance. I asked Maria if the police were still involved.

'No. There was no evidence to prosecute him. Same as last time. But he's got himself excluded from school again and referred to social services. He'll soon have been to every school this side of the Watford Gap. And *they* won't be any help.'

'Social services?'

'Yeah.'

'It sounds like Kenzie's had a difficult time. I just need to confirm that the investigation is finished, though, because if not, we would need to put therapy on hold.'

'It's finished, yeah.'

'Okay, good, that's one less thing for us to worry about.'

Maria raised her eyebrows as if to say, 'Is that it? Is that all you've got to offer me?', but I noticed that her shoulders relaxed a bit too, and she sat back from her perch on the edge of the chair, as if shifting from high alert to an ever-so slightly lesser state of alert. I hoped she was realising that I had Kenzie's interests in mind and that she could trust me to do my best for him.

Maria told me that Kenzie had first been accused of sexual assault when he was 13, but that it wasn't reported to the police because the girl retracted the allegation. She said, 'It's what these girls do these days; they want a bit of attention and so they cry rape.'

I didn't react. Instead, I wondered aloud how Kenzie had responded to the accusation.

'He didn't do it.'

'But how did he respond?'

'He said he didn't do it.'

'Was he upset?'

'I suppose so. A bit.'

'And you say there was another allegation, more recently?'

'Yeah, but there was another one last year as well.'

'So, there have been three allegations of sexual assault against Kenzie?'

'I know what you're thinking.'

'Do you…?'

'Same as everyone else – no smoke without fire.'

'I'm not thinking that, Maria. But I am wondering why Kenzie has found himself in a similar situation three times in three years and I'm wondering what I might be able to do to help him, and you, to make sense of that.'

'What *can* you do? There's never been any evidence. We get over it. We move on.'

'But it's not okay.'

'No.'

'Is this why you got in touch with me? Because of the allegations?'

'Partly that. But like I said, he's a little shit.'

I noticed her smiling and took it as a cue to lighten the mood and get alongside Maria. 'But he's *your* little shit and you're worried about him.'

'I am, yeah.'

She eased up a little and the conversation began to flow more freely. Maria told me that Kenzie had 'gone off the rails' and she doubted he would gain any qualifications. It was the autumn term of Year 11 when we first met; mock exams were looming, GCSEs were within touching distance and Kenzie didn't currently have a school place. Maria felt that he had given up on education. It sounded to me like numerous education providers might have given up on him. I wondered what he did instead, while he wasn't in school, and whether he was keeping up with his learning at home.

'You're joking.'

'I'm not.'

'I can't get him to do anything. He's in bed most of the day and out most of the night.'

'This might sound like a silly question, but I'm wondering what you'd like to be different. If I had a magic wand, which I'm afraid I don't, by the way, can you say what would change, how things would be different?' I often ask the 'magic wand' question in a first meeting.

Maria said, 'Well, he'd be in school, for a start. He'd get a couple of GCSEs, enough to go to college. He could pass them if he tried, he's not stupid.'

'Does Kenzie want to go to college?'

'He does, yeah, he wants to do animation. I think he's quite good.'

'So, he'd get a place in a school, pass his GCSEs and go to college. What else?'

'He'd get his lazy arse out of bed and help out a bit more. He does nothing.'

'What would you like him to do?'

'General stuff, you know – tidy his room, maybe push the hoover round a bit, help me with the kids.'

'The kids?'

'Yeah, I've got three younger ones, as well as Kenzie. They're 11, 9 and 3.'

'You've got your hands full.'

'I have, yeah.'

Maria told me that her middle two boys shared the same father, who she described as her best mate, while Kenzie and her youngest son each had different fathers, who had no contact with the family. She didn't seem to want to talk about them. For now, I felt I had enough of a sense of why Maria had contacted me about Kenzie without needing to delve any deeper, and Maria had relaxed enough to open up a bit, which I didn't want to jeopardise by asking more. If I was to build a relationship with Kenzie, I'd be able to build on this initial contact with Maria over time as well. I wondered what she thought about me meeting Kenzie and she said, with a smile, 'Yeah, I think you should,' which is what we arranged to happen next.

Seeing and (not) being seen

Kenzie decided he wanted to meet me online, rather than in person, which was okay by me. It's not what I prefer, but I'm happy to accept the young person's choice and explore the reasons for their preference. I logged on to the platform at the agreed time, a week or so after I'd met Kenzie's mum, and straight away there was a notification to tell me that Kenzie was waiting to join the meeting. I let him in and said hello.

'Yo.'

'Is that Kenzie?'

'It is, yeah.'

'Hello, Kenzie. I can hear you, but I can't see you.' My monitor displayed a capital 'K' against an otherwise blank, black screen.

'I've got my camera off,' he explained.

'Do you want to keep it off today?' I wondered.

'I do, yeah, if that's okay.'

'Yes, that's fine. Would you like me to keep my camera on or switch it off?'

'I don't mind.'

'Maybe I'll leave it on and then you have the choice to look at me or not.'

'Okay.'

I was reminded of the sense of withholding I'd got from Maria: the withholding of information in the initial referral and her withholding Kenzie from our initial consultation. It seemed as if that particular theme was being played out again in my first meeting with Kenzie, who had chosen to withhold his physical presence from the therapy room by opting to meet online and withhold his image from the screen by keeping his camera switched off. He'd also withheld five of the six letters of his name by displaying only his initial 'K'. In doing so, Kenzie had denied me the opportunity to witness his physical appearance – his clothes, his posture, how he moved, sat or used facial expressions, which would have provided a lot more information about him than I currently had. There was a lot I couldn't see and didn't know.

The ways in which my first meetings with Maria and Kenzie had been set up made me wonder about what might have been withheld in the family system: what might be known and not known, maybe by Kenzie; what he had been shown or told about; what he showed and told, and what might have been kept hidden. My fantasy was that this was a family with a secret. I say fantasy rather than hypothesis because, at this very early stage, all I had to base it on was an instinct, a feeling, which was tenuous but no less significant for that.

Isca Salzberger-Wittenberg, an adolescent psychotherapist influenced by Melanie Klein, said that the fantasies that we invest in a new situation are partly transferred from the past and are modified by 'inner and outer stimuli' (Salzberger-Wittenberg, 1970). In other words, as the therapeutic relationship with Kenzie developed over time, new information and behaviour (outer stimuli) would become known and new thoughts and feelings (inner stimuli) would be thought and felt, allowing my initial fantasies to change shape and either dissipate or develop into hypotheses. For now, I was acutely aware of what had been withheld, but I also needed to acknowledge what had been shared.

'It's good to hear your voice, Kenzie.'

'Thanks. You, too.'

'I'm guessing your mum told you that she came to meet me last week?'

'She did, yeah.'

'I'm wondering what she told you about our meeting?'

'Just about where you live and that you have a nice house and a nice room. And she said she thought you didn't look like your photo at first because of your hair.'

'The photo on my website?' I checked.

'Yeah.'

'Have you looked at my website?' I wondered.

'Yeah, she showed me. You look like I thought you would.'

This was fascinating. My first thoughts had been all about what I *hadn't* seen, while Kenzie's and Maria's had been about what they *had*: what my house looked like, what my room looked like, what I looked like, even what my hair looked like. There was something about the idea of seeing and (not) being seen that seemed significant and that I really wanted to explore. But not yet. First, we had to think about the therapeutic frame.

Therapeutic frame

The therapeutic frame is a symbolic boundary that contains the therapeutic relationship and helps to make therapy a safe space. It incorporates practical things like where and when therapy happens and the start and end times of sessions. It functions as a boundary to contain the creative work within it, rather like a frame around an artwork (Milner, 1952). It's important for therapeutic boundaries to be consistent, as much as possible, so that any other changes that are observed in behaviour, mood or presentation can be acknowledged as distinct. For example, younger children who are brought to and collected from sessions by different parents, or young people in care who are brought and collected by different residential workers, can present very differently in their mood, demeanour or even in the way they are dressed or whether they've been fed. I always make a request, therefore, that, if practicable, the same adult brings the child to their session at the same time each week. That way, I can more confidently attribute any differences I observe to something else.

Another important element of the therapeutic frame is confidentiality: that what happens in therapy stays in therapy, with the exceptions of supervision and matters to do with the safety of the child and others. In person-to-person therapy in the room, confidentiality is much easier to manage – control, even – than it is online. I know for certain that what is done and said in the therapy room is only witnessed by the people doing the doing and saying. Therapy online doesn't carry the same certainties. In the real world, I know that what I'm doing and saying at my end isn't being witnessed. In the online world, I use a platform with high levels of security. I use a log-in and authentication process that provides a unique link for each client, every session, which enables them to access an online waiting room, where they wait until I invite them in. This is a bit like them knocking at the door at the start of their in-person session and waiting for me to open it. At the end of each session, I delete any online chat (text), as well as the meeting link and the invitation, so that I'm not saving any data whatsoever related to the session.

What I'm saying is, I do all that I can to maintain privacy and confidentiality, in both the real and the online world. An important difference is that, with online therapy, I inform the young person and their parent or carer that it is their responsibility to arrange a private space where they will not be disturbed, interrupted or overheard during their session, and I check in with them about this every week. But I have no control over it; all I have is their word. I checked in with Kenzie.

'Before we get started, Kenzie, I just wanted to let you know that I'm in my office on my own, and this is where I will always be when I speak to you online, so I'm not being overheard and I won't be interrupted.'

'Okay.'

'What about you?'

'What do you mean?'

'I just want to check that you are somewhere on your own, that feels private to talk.'

'Yeah.'

'That's good. It's hard for me to know that when we're online, so I wanted to check.'

'Yeah, I'm on my own.'

'That's good. I wonder if there's anything you want to check out with me, Kenzie?'

'No.'

'Okay. Maybe you could tell me how you feel about the idea of talking to me – a therapist, I mean.'

'I'm not sure. It was my mum's idea.'

'Okay. Why do you think *she* wanted you to talk to me?'

'Because of what happened…'

'Because of what happened?'

'Yeah. She probably told you.'

'She told me some stuff when we met. But I wonder if you can say what you mean. I'd like to hear it from you.' It's always important for me to hear it from the young person themselves.

'About the rape.'

'The rape?'

'Yeah. What the girl said I did.'

'Your mum did mention that, yes.' There was no point pretending that she hadn't, no point *withholding* the fact that I knew.

I commented, 'It sounds like you've had a tough time.'

'Yeah, it's been shit.'

'I'm sorry to hear that.'

'That's okay.'

'It's not okay though, is it? Like you said, it's shit.'

'Yeah.'

'Can you tell me about how shit it's been?'

'Not really. I don't want to talk about it. I don't mean to be rude,' he added.

'It's okay, Kenzie, and it's not rude. I'm pleased you were able to say no. It's difficult to talk about private stuff when we've only just met.' I cringed internally, worried that I'd pushed too far already. 'What would you like us to talk about instead?'

'I dunno.'

'What about school?'

'I don't go to school.'

I'd put my foot in it again. I knew that he didn't go to school, but I hadn't kept it in mind, and I'd relied on a lazy, stock question – you don't want to talk about the hard stuff, okay, let's talk about something more trivial like school.

'Yes, I know, your mum told me that too. Is there any news about when you might start back?'

'I don't think so. No one's said anything to me.'

'How is that for you, not being at school?'

'It's okay, actually. Better.'
'Better how?'
'I dunno. It just is.'
'You sound quite chilled. I wonder if it's more chilled not being at school.'
'Definitely.'
'It's your GCSE year, isn't it?'
'Yeah.'
'And what comes next?'
'Hopefully I'll go to college.'

After a stilted start, Kenzie seemed to come alive as he talked about his passion and talent for drawing – he became animated once he started talking about animation. So much so that this is what we spoke about for the remainder of the session. Before we ended, I suggested he might like to show me some of his work in our next session, as it was something we could look at together online. I thought it might be a nice way for me to show I was interested in him and a way for Kenzie to share something of himself in a less intimate way than showing himself. He said he'd think about it.

I'd been primed to meet a boy who was three times accused of sexual assault, currently excluded from school and described as a lazy, out-of-control little shit who needed sorting out. I ended the first session, despite having spent it looking at a blank screen, with a sense of a passionate and talented young man, full of life and potential. The blank screen provided an interesting context, because another way of thinking about what was hidden or not seen was that all other distractions were removed, so that all I had to focus on was Kenzie's spoken word. I was excited to discover more.

Process and content

The following week, I was feeling very different to how I'd felt in week one as I waited to meet Kenzie for his second session. I don't usually read back over my notes from previous sessions – not that I had many notes to read yet. Instead, I try to meet each client for every session with as little expectation as possible. As I wait, though, particularly if I have to wait very long, thoughts start to emerge, and it's important to acknowledge them. When I'm kept waiting after the session is due to begin, my first thought is usually, 'Have I got the time wrong?' If it's an online session, it's 'Did I send the correct link to the correct email address?' Once I'm sure that I haven't made a mistake, I start to wonder about the lateness, which is what happened here, as I waited for Kenzie to join me for his second session. At first, I wondered if I'd put him off, perhaps by inviting him to tell me about the accusations made against him, or by being clumsy in asking about school. Then I remembered how he'd seemed to settle as the session progressed and how we'd begun to build a rapport in discussing his passion for animation. I hoped I'd be able to explore this with him further and get to know him through his art, which must, I thought, be autobiographical in some way. I think anything that is created must say something about its creator, be that drawing, painting, sculpture or writing. I acknowledge that my writing – what I say, how I say it and what I leave out – must also say something about me. When I recalled my conversation with Kenzie, I realised that he had told me he made computer animations and pencil sketches, the *how* rather than the *what*. This led me to think about the distinction between process (how) and content (what), both in relation to art and in therapeutic terms.

The content of art is the picture: a landscape, portrait or cartoon. The content of therapy is what happens in the room, such as what is said or done and by whom. The process of art is the way the picture is created – maybe the medium that's used: paint, pencil or collage. The process of therapy is the relationship within and between the two (or more) people who come together for the purpose of therapy. When I was training, I wrote copious notes after each session, documenting the content and trying laboriously to record every word that was uttered and berating myself if I missed something out, which I inevitably did. Over time, with the help of my tutors and supervisors, I realised that therapy notes are often referred to as 'process recordings' for a very good reason: they record the process rather than the content. By process, I mean the thoughts, feelings, fantasies and hypotheses that I experience during and after the session. Again, as a novice psychotherapist, I remember finding it difficult to process in the moment – all my attention was focused on doing; I didn't have the capacity to think about what I was thinking and notice what I was feeling all at the same time – and most of my processing happened when I reflected on the sessions afterwards.

As I reflected on Kenzie's first session afterwards, I thought it was interesting that he'd shared his process with me, rather than his content, and I wondered if that might be something to consider when (if?) we met again for therapy. Psychotherapists, particularly newly qualified ones, can feel a pressure to say something clever and useful in order to illustrate, to their client and to themselves, that they are doing something clever and useful. I think this is a similar pressure to the one I'd felt to write lengthy, detailed notes: to demonstrate, if only to myself, that something useful had taken place. While it can be helpful to document our thinking and share it with clients, sometimes it's enough just to feel the feeling or think the thought and process it without verbalisation. That way, our clients can have 'an emotional experience rather than an intellectual one' (Gray, 2014).

As the time ticked by and Kenzie remained absent from his second session, I wondered about his experience of session one – had it been an emotional experience for him and, if so, was the experience good enough? I also began to wonder about his wider emotional experiences, in the family generally and in response to the allegations made against him specifically. I remembered that, when I'd asked his mother about his response to the accusations, she'd struggled to answer the question, telling me instead that he didn't *do* it. Even when I'd offered her an emotion-type prompt, by wondering if he was upset, she'd found it difficult to answer and said only that she supposed so. It was as if she was saying that was how someone would be *supposed* to respond, rather than how Kenzie actually did react. I wondered if she'd really noticed how he processed the news. Thinking in terms of content and process, my meeting with Maria had been full of content, which made me wonder about her capacity to process her own feelings and to hold Kenzie emotionally. One of the primary tasks of a parent 'is to learn how to contain the baby' (Brazelton & Cramer, 1990, p.114). I was left wondering about the extent to which Maria had managed that in Kenzie's early years and beyond.

I spent the therapeutic hour thinking about and processing my very different experiences with Kenzie and Maria. Towards the end of the 50 minutes, I sent a message to Maria saying I was sorry not to have met with Kenzie for his session and that I hoped everything was okay. The response I received said, 'He forgot. Can he video-call you tomorrow?', demonstrating either an inability or an unwillingness to hold in mind Kenzie's therapy (perhaps Kenzie himself?) and/or the therapeutic boundaries. I sent a short, polite response stating that it was not possible to meet tomorrow, but that I looked forward to hearing from Kenzie next week, and I re-stated the date and time of the session. If therapists agree to *ad hoc* sessions, or requests to start early or end late, we alter the therapeutic frame and threaten the containing function of therapy. As Gray states, if clients find that the framework is changed to suit them, they 'will be worried about the therapist's ability to contain powerful emotions' (Gray, 2014, p.45).

I'm certain that Maria and Kenzie would not have been consciously worried, but at some level they would sense that the boundaries were loose, which would threaten their sense of safety and containment. This is akin to the child who asks the parent for something – say, a packet of sweets. The parent says no, the child asks again, the parent says no, the child pushes and whines and the parent feels forced to acquiesce. In the moment, the child is delighted that they got the sweets, but what they learn from this encounter is that parents don't mean what they say, that 'no' can mean 'yes', which is confusing, and that boundaries are moveable. So, what becomes internalised is a sense of non-containment. If I'd agreed to speak to Kenzie the next day, instead of on the day we'd arranged, he and Maria might have been pleased not to have to wait; I would have been pleased to speak to him too, but they would have got a sense, like the child of the acquiescing parent, that I was unable to contain them. Remember, this was a family with a theme of withholding, so holding the boundary felt especially important. I didn't give them what they said they wanted, but I believe that I did provide what was needed.

Pushing the boundaries

The following week, Kenzie joined the meeting on time and apologised for forgetting the previous session. Like the first time, he didn't have his camera turned on and, like before, I checked that this was a conscious decision. It was. I told him that there was no need to apologise for missing the session; he hadn't done anything wrong. I also let him know that I'd spent the time keeping him in mind, and I wondered what he'd been doing instead.

'I can't remember.'
'Something that took your attention.'
'Yeah, must have been.'
'I'm wondering how you've been spending your week. What have you been up to?'

'Not much… Watching YouTube… Drawing… Hanging out with my mates…'

'So, some relaxing stuff and some creative stuff, and some time on your own and some time with your mates.'

'Yeah, I suppose.'

'That sounds like a nice balance. What do you like to watch on YouTube.'

'The usual.'

'I don't know what "the usual" is for you, Kenzie.'

'Fails, blunders. There's also some animators I follow on Insta who post content.'

'That sounds like a balance too, between fails and successes.'

'Yeah, I hadn't thought of it like that.'

'It makes me wonder about *your* fails and successes?'

He said, 'I don't have any successes.'

'I find that difficult to believe,' I countered.

'It's true.'

'It's easier for you to think about your fails?'

'Yeah, there's plenty of them.'

'I'm sorry to hear you say that about yourself.'

'It's what everyone says.'

'Everyone?'

'Yeah.'

'They talk about your fails.'

'Yeah.'

'That's a shame. I wonder why that's what they focus on.'

'Mud sticks.'

'What do you mean by that?'

'It's what my mum says.'

I remembered the other phrase Maria had said to me – 'There's no smoke without fire', which seemed to have a similar connotation – and asked, 'I'm wondering what you think she means by mud sticks?'

'That I'm a little shit and a useless fucker.'

I heard a noise through the computer speaker that didn't sound like Kenzie. 'I heard what you said, Kenzie, but I also heard another noise in the background, like maybe another voice.'

Silence.

'It makes me wonder if there's someone else there with you?'

'Errr, no…'

'You're in the room on your own?'

Silence.

The noise I'd heard sounded like something between a loud gasp and a muffled laugh. The word that came to mind, which is old-fashioned and not one I'd usually use, was 'guffaw'. It made me feel uneasy.

There was a silence of about 30 seconds, which felt like a really long time, and then a woman's voice said, 'Hi, Jeanine, sorry.'

'Maria?' I enquired.

'Yes, it's me.'

'You're in the room with Kenzie?'

'Yes, but I promise I'm not listening,' she insisted.

'It's really important that Kenzie's sessions are private and that you can make space for him to access therapy without being overheard.' If I sounded punitive, it was because I felt punitive.

'Yes, sorry. I'll go in the other room.'

I'd explained the importance of privacy and confidentiality, and I felt tricked and betrayed. I'd been kept in the dark, with the camera switched off, so that Maria had been able to intrude into the session without me knowing. While it was important to notice my feelings – tricked, betrayed, intruded upon, kept in the dark, not-knowing – I wondered how Kenzie felt.

'How come your mum was in the room?'

'I dunno. She said she wasn't listening, though.'

'I think it's kind of impossible not to listen, don't you?'

'Maybe.'

'I heard her make a noise when you mentioned her.'

'Yeah, I think her ears pricked up when she heard her name.'

'I'm wondering why she was there?' I pressed.

'She asked me if I wanted her to go out.'

'And you said no?'

'I said I didn't mind.'

'And so she took that to mean it was okay to stay?'

'Yeah.'

'In *your* therapy session.'

'Yeah.'

I wondered to myself about not saying no meaning yes, and I wondered aloud how much privacy Kenzie felt that he had at home.

'Not much, really. I have to share a room with my brother. It's a bit pants, to be honest. That's why I go out so much when he's home.'

'I think it's important to have some space and time of your own that feels private.'

'So do I!'

'And it's difficult not to have that. Especially when you're 16.'

'Exactly. But my mum doesn't see it like that. She's got her nose in everything.'

'In your business, you mean?'

'Yeah.'

'I think it's hard for mums of 16-year-olds too.' I didn't want Kenzie to feel I was colluding with him against his mum. 'She really cares about you, and it sounds as if she has her hands full and that the house is quite crowded.'

'I suppose.'

I also wanted him to know that I was beginning to understand what it was like for him, so I repeated, 'But it's still important for you to have some privacy.' And I tentatively added, 'Perhaps we can think about how we can make therapy a private space for you? Perhaps you'd like to think about coming here.'

'Yeah, I'll think about it. Thanks.'

After the session, I received an email from Maria, apologising for being in the room and assuring me it wouldn't happen again. She seemed anxious to placate me, but I wondered what else she might be anxious about: possibly about what Kenzie might share with me, or what might become un-hidden? Why else would she need to eavesdrop on his therapy session? She also said in the email that there was 'some other stuff' she thought I should know. We had already arranged to meet in week six, to think about how therapy was going for Kenzie and whether he wanted to carry on. I asked if Maria felt the 'other stuff' could wait until then and she said it could.

Being in synch

Kenzie attended his next two online sessions on time and on his own. He switched on his camera and scanned the room to prove to me that there was no one else there. This demonstrated that he had internalised the importance of keeping the boundary, but also, more significantly perhaps, it illustrated that he was letting himself be seen by me. I wondered what else might be revealed or become un-hidden or un-withheld. He said his mum had offered to walk the dogs, so that she wasn't in the house during his sessions and couldn't be tempted to listen in. Evidently, Maria was thinking about the boundaries too.

It was nice to see Kenzie. He was a pleasant-looking, well-presented young man, who seemed to take pride in his appearance: his hair was styled, and his clothes looked clean and ironed. The words that came to my mind were that he looked like someone who took care of himself. The other thing I noticed about Kenzie was that his skin was darker than Maria's and I wondered if he was mixed race. Maria hadn't mentioned it; perhaps that was something else that had been withheld. If so, I wondered why. Kenzie spent the sessions talking about and showing me his animations. They were fabulous in terms of the detail, and his talent was obvious. I found myself making lots of congratulatory, impressed-sounding noises, because I was very struck by his skill and his dedication to something that clearly took hours to create. But I had a sense it might be too much for Kenzie. He seemed pleased, but a bit awkward, as if what I was saying to and about him, or how I was saying it, felt unfamiliar and uncomfortable.

I remembered Maria's description of her son as 'a little shit' – while it was said affectionately, it wasn't complimentary – and noted that Kenzie would have picked up on that and internalised it. He'd told me of his sense that his mum thought he was 'a useless fucker' and his description of her as having 'her nose in everything' – which sounded mistrustful and intrusive. I also recalled the comments about mud sticking and there being no smoke without fire, which felt so out of synch with the young man I was starting to get to know. I began to hypothesise about what Maria's attunement with the baby Kenzie once was, because that's where in-synch or out-of-synch-ness begins.

Mothers (usually) learn the rhythms of their babies by watching, responding and prolonging their attention. They look for cues, such as smiling or crying, moving towards or away from, and they match their responses accordingly, so that the rhythms of the mother become synchronised with those of the baby (Brazelton & Cramer, 1990). This is a rewarding experience for both parties in the mother–infant dyad: the baby learns that s/he is loved, known and understood, which forms the foundations of its capacity to love, know and understand her/himself; the mother learns that she is loved by her baby, and is inclined to keep loving her baby back because it feels nice to be loved. In this way, the beginnings of our earliest attachments are formed – attachments that go on to shape all the relationships that follow.

According to the psychologist, psychiatrist and psychoanalyst John Bowlby (1979), there are both short- and long-term benefits of early attachment. The most immediate short-term benefit is that of survival: if a baby isn't loved and attended to by a loving and attentive mother, it will die. Those relentless cries of a 'needy' baby are expressing its deepest fears. As Melanie Klein observed, what the baby is communicating in its cries is, 'I need you, I must have you all the time… I cannot survive without you' (Salzberger-Wittenberg, 1970, p.57). Longer-term benefits of attachment are to do with the way that they shape our relationships through childhood and adolescence and into adulthood. Bowlby suggested that babies develop an internal model that is based on the attachment with their mother, which gives them a sense of self and is a prototype for all other relationships, including intimate relationships. So, if a baby develops a secure early attachment, their model of self is of being lovable and they are more likely to go on to form secure intimate relationships. If, on the other hand, a baby has a less than good-enough experience of attachment, perhaps because its mother is out of synch, preoccupied, inconsistent or absent, it develops a negative sense of self. In future relationships, those 'babies' might be overly dependent on others and preoccupied with intimacy, perhaps to make up for what they lacked in infancy; or they might avoid intimacy and keep themselves to themselves, because they have learnt that they can't depend on others to meet their needs (Bartholomew & Horowitz, 1991). I had a sense of Kenzie as an avoidant kind of 'baby', out-of-synch, avoidant of intimacy, and taking care of himself. The first therapy review would put all of my fantasies into context.

Ghosts of the past

Maria arrived a few minutes early for the therapy review. As with the initial consultation, she came alone. I usually encourage young people who I'm working with to attend their therapy reviews for the simple reason that they are *their* therapy reviews and I have a belief that they should be privy to what is being thought and said about them. Some young people opt out, for a number of reasons, and I respect their choice to do so. Maria was keen to talk to me without Kenzie present and Kenzie was keen not to come. He'd decided to 'take a break' from therapy; perhaps it was beginning to feel intimate and perhaps he wasn't ready for intimacy yet. I respected his decision. I hoped he'd internalised a good-enough experience of psychotherapy to be able to come back if and when the time was right for him. Before ending, I asked Kenzie if there was anything in particular that he did or didn't want me to share, and we agreed that I would focus on the process rather than the content of his therapy: how he'd begun to share things with me, show me his art and show me himself. I was pleased that Maria agreed with me that we should still meet, to mark the end of her son's engagement in therapy. I clocked that she was early and sensed some anxiety, the source of which became immediately apparent.

'There's something I didn't tell you before that I think you should know.' She seemed in a hurry to get it out.

'I'm listening,' I assured her.

'I was raped.'

'Oh, Maria. I'm so sorry to hear that.'

'By Kenzie's father.'

I have an expressive face that can't hide how I feel, and I know that my eyes widened and my eyebrows raised.

Maria registered my alarm, but continued, 'We'd been hanging out for a bit. He was okay. Well, not really okay, but you know…'

'Okay but not-okay?' I wondered.

'Well, more not-okay as it turned out. He was mates with some people I knew. I didn't know him that well. He was older, early 20s. I was only 17. He was good looking. Exotic. His mother was from Bangladesh. I realised he liked me, but I wasn't sure.'

'You weren't sure how you felt about that?'

'I wasn't sure how I felt about *him*, but I knew how I felt about him liking me. It sounds awful, but I suppose I was flattered.'

'It doesn't sound awful, it sounds ordinary. It must have been nice to feel that a good-looking, older man had noticed you.'

'I don't think I led him on or anything. Or maybe I did. I hardly spoke to him, really. We never went out or anything.'

'It sounds like you're trying to make sense of what happened to you; work out whether you were responsible.'

'That's what I've been trying to do for the last 17 years!'

'I don't know what happened, Maria, and I don't need to know. But what I do know is that you are absolutely not responsible for being raped. Kenzie's father is wholly responsible for what he did to you.'

I noticed a tear begin to form in her eye, but quick as a flash it was sucked back in and she was back in control.

'He doesn't know,' she whispered.

'He doesn't know?' I asked.
'He doesn't know he got me pregnant.'
'I'm wondering if Kenzie knows.'
'No.'

Suddenly, the themes and fantasies I'd been holding in mind over the few months since Maria made contact started to join up. The withholding of information in the referral, withholding Kenzie from our initial consultation, Kenzie withholding his physical presence by opting to work online and withholding his appearance by switching off the camera. I remembered his words in our first session, 'No one's said anything to me,' and my fantasy about a family secret, which had now been revealed to me and which no one had said anything to Kenzie about. I recalled feeling tricked, betrayed, intruded upon and kept in the dark, as well as all the experiences I'd had of not-knowing. I also remembered the first conversation I'd had with Maria. One of her opening statements was 'mud sticks'. It struck me now that this was historic mud, mud from the rape that had stuck to Maria and been passed on to Kenzie and stuck to him. That's what she'd said when she'd told me about the allegations of sexual assault that had been made against her son, which had precipitated the referral to therapy. She'd also told me 'It's not the first time', and I wondered now whether she'd been thinking about her own experience. I wondered if, when she'd said 'They cry rape' about Kenzie's accusers, she'd been projecting onto them the way she thought others might perceive her. I also wondered whether she'd told anyone about what had happened to her and I remembered her saying, 'We get over it. We move on.' She'd also said, 'He's gonna end up locked up,' and I reflected on the locked-up, muddy secret that Maria had carried for 17 years – Kenzie's entire life – and wondered if the man who raped her had ever been locked up for his crime.

Those three small words 'I was raped' carried so much meaning: for me, for Maria and, even though he had no conscious awareness of it, for Kenzie too. He was a young man who had been conceived through rape, who hadn't been told, but had somehow got caught up in a repeated pattern of allegations of sexual assault, where not saying no could be interpreted as yes. Freud proposed an innate tendency to repeat both pleasurable and painful experiences, which he called the repetition compulsion (Freud, 1920). Could it be that these compulsions could be re-enacted across generations? And if the struggle between love (of self and other) and hate (of self and other) is inherent, could it be that baby Kenzie had internalised a sense of himself as 'bad' – a little shit, a useless fucker – because he was born out of 'badness'? And what about the literal meaning of 'useless fucker' in the context of rape? Kenzie's biological father was the worst type of useless fucker: he was an abusive fucker.

Selma Fraiberg, a child psychoanalyst and social worker, coined the term 'ghosts in the nursery' to refer to the repetition of the past in the present (Fraiberg et al., 1975). Fraiberg's ghosts include the parents' own traumatic experiences and the ways in which they themselves were parented, which come into play in the present narrative – the ghost story, as it were. Kenzie's ghost story began with a rape and that terrifying, abusive, intrusive ghost must have been omnipresent throughout Maria's pregnancy, right up to the present day, casting a dark shadow over the mother–child relationship and obscuring, if not obliterating, Kenzie – the actual, in-his-own-right Kenzie – from view. But how? How can an experience that happened to someone else, before Kenzie was even born, get re-enacted in him/by him years later? I don't have a definitive answer, but I and many others have witnessed it time and again, and it's an area of ongoing research. If eye colour, hair colour and a talent for tap dancing can be inherited, why not experiences? I explore the theme of ghosts in the nursery in more detail in Chapter 7.

Child and family psychiatrist John Byng-Hall has shared his observations of working with families who repeat destructive patterns almost as if they are following a predetermined script. But he also suggests that repetition can be the 'launching pad for change' (Byng-Hall, 1995). I would develop that statement further by saying it is the *acknowledgment* of family scripts and 'ghosts in the nursery' that precipitates change. I wonder if, at some level, Maria had sent Kenzie to therapy on her behalf – he'd said 'It was my mum's idea because of what happened' – to begin the process of acknowledgement vicariously through him, just as he had been acting out her story vicariously during his adolescence. Either way, they had found their way to where we were now and I had every faith in them to keep going on their own, together, and maybe, in time, with further therapeutic support. Was Kenzie's fate mapped out at the moment of conception, and was it inevitable that the past would play out in the present? I don't believe so. In my experience, history doesn't always repeat itself, but quite often it rhymes.

3
Lessons in love

Della lives in the shadow of her mad sister and is always 'fucking around' with boys and weed and alcohol, which makes her feel bad. Can therapy help her to improve her sense of self-worth and decide to make some changes?

. . . .

The first time I met them, Della and her father were sharing an energy drink as they waited for me to open the door, as if they were mates rather than parent and child. Della's appearance was striking. I knew she was 16, but I didn't think she looked it. She seemed slight and underweight, giving the impression of a pre-pubescent girl. Her make-up was heavy and dark and seemed to mask poor skin. Her hair was dyed blue-black. Her appearance was the epitome of what might be called goth or emo.

I had received a brief psychotherapy referral from Della's father, and we'd had a telephone conversation by way of introduction. He had brought her to the first session, but Della decided she wanted to come in on her own, which surprised me, given the apparent closeness I'd witnessed. After we'd made our introductions and I'd explained the boundaries of the therapeutic contract, I invited Della to tell me in her own words why she had come to therapy. This was the only cue she needed to talk incessantly throughout the entire first session.

Della's story began with descriptions of lots of movement within and between the family. Her parents were divorced and she lived with dad, while her older sister Kiki had moved between their mother's home and an adolescent psychiatric hospital. Della displayed no emotional affect as she described her family, and I wondered aloud how she felt about all the changes. She shrugged and said, 'I just get on with it.' I also noticed a lack of emotional response to meeting me: there'd been no sign of apprehension or anxiety and no sense of her needing to settle in; she just started talking. I thought of Della's words as filling the space, rather than engaging in dialogue with me. The only way I could comment or join in was if I interrupted her, which made me feel clumsy and awkward.

As this was the only apparent feeling response that I was aware of in the room, it seemed significant. It's important to feel and to acknowledge the feeling. As Redland states, 'In our line of work, we can't just think and do, we must feel' (Redland, 2020, p.131). I wondered if my feeling communicated something about Della's own experiences in the world. That happens in therapy sometimes, when a feeling isn't really my feeling at all, it's a clue about how the other person might be feeling but perhaps isn't aware of or isn't able to say. This is an example of reciprocal transference, where we carry stuff on behalf of the client. Perhaps my sense of being clumsy and awkward in the way we were communicating was telling me something about communication in Della's family; perhaps it, too, felt clumsy and awkward. Perhaps, in order to join in, she had to interrupt. I'd already heard about a mentally unwell sister, who I assumed took up a lot of space in the family, even when she wasn't physically there.

Della presented a potted history of her parents' marital breakdown and their numerous relationships since, which mostly seemed to include violence and betrayal of some sort or other. It seemed that she knew a lot of detail, including her father's employment of prostitutes, and I felt concerned about the boundaries between Della and each of her parents. I wondered aloud what effect she felt her experience of her parents' relationships had on her own and she told me, with an apparent lack of self-consciousness, about a series of sexual encounters. She identified herself as the 'okay for now' girl, which meant that boys would 'talk to her', by which she meant 'have sex with her', until someone 'better' came along. When I wondered why she accepted this role and whether, perhaps, it felt familiar, she said, 'Kiki is the special one.'

'Your sister?' I checked.

'Yeah.'

'She's more special than you?'

'Yeah. She gets all the attention.'

'From your parents?'

'From everyone.'

'I'm wondering where that leaves you?'

'No one pays any attention to me. So I just fuck around.'

'Fuck around how?'

'You know, with boys and stuff.'
'And stuff…?'
'Yeah.'
'And no one notices?'
'Not really. They wouldn't notice if I was gone.'
'Can I check what you mean by gone, Della?'
'Dead.'

It seemed there was a narrative in the family, at least as far as Della told it, that her sister Kiki was the special one who got all the attention, which left Della taking up the position of the bad/fucking-around one who didn't. It was too early to hypothesise about where this narrative had originated, but it seemed clear that Della had internalised a sense of herself as unnoticeable, unspecial and worthless. I also hypothesised that Della might be acting out sexually with lots of 'notice me' type behaviour as a consequence of her need to be noticed at home not being met. Apparent 'bad', risky or unhealthy behaviour is often the consequence of an unmet need.

Della described, without any apparent affect or emotion, a litany of encounters that sounded abusive, including betrayal by her best friend and mistreatment by several 'boys'. She seemed to dive straight in and trust people before getting to know them – just as she had dived straight into talking to me – and was repeatedly hurt and abused as a consequence. One particular incident that she recalled involved a boy of 18 who had sex with her and then threw a towel in her direction and told her to 'clean yourself up before you go'. She didn't think that was particularly unusual and didn't seem to think she deserved anything more. She recited a long list of her 'faults', including drug-taking, excessive alcohol consumption and under-age sex, as if to illustrate her 'badness' and worthlessness to me. I was struck by the way Della told me so much intimate detail about her sexual life within minutes of meeting me and with an apparent lack of self-awareness. This seemed to me to parallel her life outside the therapy room, as a person's presentation within it so often does.

I suggested to Della that we could meet three more times, four sessions in total, and then decide about whether to continue meeting or not. We could think of this as a kind of assessment period, where I could get to know more about Della and what she wanted from therapy, and she could experience the kind of therapy I offer and decide whether she found it helpful. I think it's important to mark out an assessment period, to give both me and a potential client an opportunity to decide if we're a good-enough match, without any expectations about commitment to a long-term relationship. This seemed particularly important with Della, given my sense of her experience of relationships.

That first session left me feeling heavy and flat. There was a lot of work to do to make sense of Della's sense of self, but, despite her agreeing to my suggestion, I wasn't sure she would come back.

Therapy assessment

Della did come back. Again, her father brought her to the session, a few minutes late. Again, they seemed 'matey' in the way they interacted. When I have a sense of parents and children as 'friends' rather than parents and children, or when a young person or a parent describes the other as their 'best friend' – usually with a big grin, as if that's not only a good thing, but the *best thing ever* – it always raises my concern. It begs the question, if your mother or father is your best friend, who is parenting you? In the case of Della's family, I noticed that I was asking myself this question, and saved it for another time.

As Della moved away from her father to follow me into the therapy room, she asked him to look after her phone, which struck me as incredibly unusual. There are few 16 year olds willing to be separated from their phone at all, and fewer still who would willingly hand it over to their father! I wondered about the potential symbolism of Della handing over something personal and precious to her dad. There was seemingly much to explore in the father/daughter relationship, and I stored that thought away too. During every therapeutic encounter, I'm in constant dialogue with my own thoughts, noticing them, processing them, sometimes sharing them, but more often storing them away for later examination (Gray, 2014). Once we were in the privacy of the therapy room, I asked Della how she felt about coming to the second session.

She said, 'I didn't want to.'
'I'd been wondering about that.'
'Had you?'
'Yes.'
'Why?'
'Well, because you told me so much in our first session, and I wondered what it would feel like to come back to it, to come back to me, knowing that I know.'

'That's why I didn't want to come.'
'Because of what you told me?'
'Because it made me feel sad.'

It seemed as if Della hadn't considered in the first session what it would be like to meet me again, once I knew something intimate about her. I thought about the similarities between this and her one-night stands, where she shared intimate parts of her physical self during a first meeting and then didn't go back. I encouraged Della to share her thoughts about wanting to come – because she *had* come after all, so there must at least be a part of her that wanted to – and about not wanting to come.

'I'm not mental. It's not like I *need* to come.'
'Yet here you are.'
She ignored the fact and said again, 'But I'm not mental.'
'Can you tell me about your understanding of mental, Della?'
'Like my sister.'
'You think of her as mental?'
'Er, yeah. Because she is. She's proper mental. She got locked up!'
'Kiki is so "mental" that she went into hospital.'
'Exactly!'
'So,' I wondered, 'you're telling me that you're not the same as Kiki? You're not "proper mental"?'
'God no! I'm nothing like her. She's insane! Like, *literally* insane!'
'Literally insane?'
'Absolutely!'
'I see.'

I saw a bit. I saw that Della was distancing herself from her sister and from mental illness, splitting off the 'madness' and locating it in her sister. She changed the subject, as if that topic was done and dusted.

'And I can't come here on Fridays.' I'd offered her an after-school slot on a Friday afternoon.
'Okay. Why's that?'
'It's practically the weekend. I'm not going to therapy at the weekend!'
'Quite right! The weekend is when you have your freedom, get to do your own thing. We can look at changing the time of your session. I'm sorry, I didn't think of that.'

I think I played it right, but Della eyed me suspiciously, as if my words might be a trap. I wondered to myself about the link she might be making between therapy and the school week, as if these were things that she felt she was made to do rather than things she could choose to do or not do for herself. I was thinking too about the sexual activities she didn't seem to have much agency over, the things she maybe felt she was made to do, but it felt too early in our therapeutic relationship to voice the link out loud. I was wary of becoming someone else who might 'make' her do something she wasn't comfortable doing, or someone who she felt would 'make' her talk about stuff she wasn't ready to talk about. I tried to move things along by checking in that I'd understood what Della had told me so far.

'So, you're not mental, you don't like the Friday evening slot, which we can look at changing, and yet here you are, you came. I'm impressed.'

'Thanks.' She raised a smile.

'Can you say why you came?'

'I do want things to be different.'

'Okay. And…?'

'And coming here might stop me being so bad. But mainly it's because of my dad.'

'Your dad?'

'Yeah.'

She didn't elaborate and I chose not to ask her to. Instead, I filed away the fact that Della had told me she was coming to therapy because of her dad, and I wondered what that might mean – that she was coming because her dad wanted her to, or perhaps to explore something about their relationship. Time would tell.

During the remainder of the assessment sessions, Della continued to talk freely, and was able to meet my gentle challenges, which felt promising. She told me about strategies she had used to feel better, which included writing lyrics and keeping a diary, as well as more destructive methods such as self-injury, alcohol and sex. This led us to thinking about if and how therapy might help. Della told me that Kiki often read her diary and notebooks and used her words to blackmail her, threatening to tell their parents what she'd written if she didn't do what she wanted, so that the only outcome was negative. She didn't talk to her mum about stuff. Sometimes she talked to her dad.

I shared my thoughts about how therapy might help Della to open up a dialogue that might be different, helpful even, and how it might feel unusual for her in that I would have no agenda and wouldn't take what she said or did personally. Della fell silent, which was rare, and appeared to reflect on what I'd said. The silence was broken by her saying again that no one was nice to her and why was I being nice when she didn't deserve it. I'd begun to recognise this as a default position. I had no doubt it was a familiar sense of self, but I also wondered if it was being used defensively. It was as if Della was saying, 'If I keep reminding us both that I'm worthless and that nobody cares about me, you won't care about me either and I won't have to risk forming a relationship with you.' I noticed again that, when Della spoke about being treated badly, she showed no emotional affect, as if she was immune to the difficult feelings and the abusive treatment. In contrast, she seemed to experience me with an element of suspicion, as if she couldn't work out why I wasn't treating her the same way she felt everyone else did.

In the final assessment session, Della announced that she didn't *want* to carry on coming to therapy, but that she *would* carry on because it was something she probably *should* do. I acknowledged her understandable ambivalence about embarking on psychotherapy, that coming here must feel difficult in light of her experience of her sister's mental illness and her own thoughts and feelings about what that meant. I also acknowledged her courage in being willing to give it a go. Embarking on therapy is always courageous.

Making a relationship

In our first session following the assessments, Della told me she was back with her ex-boyfriend Jimmy, and that they were officially an item again. I thought this was interesting timing – perhaps she was telling me she was in a relationship with someone more special than me and that our relationship could never be as special as that one. Or maybe she was saying that she didn't need me because she had Jimmy. Or perhaps talking about the 'special new relationship' with Jimmy was a way of acknowledging our new and (potentially) special relationship. I've noticed that the therapeutic relationship often changes shape and feel following completion of the assessment period and I think young people recognise that too. I encouraged Della to tell me more about Jimmy, but kept in mind that she might be communicating something of her sense of our relationship too.

She said she really missed him when they weren't together and couldn't imagine ever breaking up with him again. She was clearly smitten – for the time being, at least. Della described how the relationship had developed from hanging out to flirting to being boyfriend and girlfriend. It sounded ordinary, age appropriate and fun, in stark contrast to Della's other experiences with boys that I'd heard about. When I said this, Della told me she had decided not to have sex with Jimmy when they were together before, because she was only 15 and he didn't want to break the law. I clocked that *he'd* made the decision not to have sex, although she had presented it as if it was *her* decision – the familiar theme of other people deciding things for Della and her seeming not to notice or not be bothered. I wondered about her sense of self as separate; it was as if she became merged with the people she was in relationship with and got swallowed up by them and disappeared.

    As if to prove the wonderfulness of Jimmy, Della went on to tell me about a contrasting experience with a different ex-boyfriend who had 'made me put my hand down his trousers on the day we met'. I commented that it seemed difficult, sometimes, for Della to take control of how she was in a relationship and to set boundaries that she was comfortable with. She said she regretted having sex with boys and going too far in the past, but she said this in a self-punishing rather than a reflective way, as if it was her fault, and as if she believed that she was inherently 'bad'.

    Della seemed vulnerable in her relationships and totally without any sense of autonomy. The other person was always the one to decide when and how it started, when and how it ended and what happened in between. Her relationships began when someone else instigated them and ended when someone else cheated on her or dumped her. I hoped that therapy could offer a different experience of how a relationship could be. I commented that Della had already begun to express how she wanted it to be here in negotiating the change of day. She told me it felt different to her previous experience of counselling, which she hadn't liked, but went along with. I reiterated how important it was that Della didn't 'go along with' things here, that she was in charge of what we did and didn't talk about and how long we continued to meet, even how much of each 50-minute session she stayed for – absolutely everything about *her* therapy was *her* choice. She looked confused, and I wondered if perhaps she didn't know how to be in control. I asked how she'd been since we last met.

    'I've been okay. Jimmy's a good influence.'

'In what way?'

'I haven't been drunk or high. And I've been to all my lessons because he wants me to do well at school.'

I repeated, 'Because *Jimmy* wants you to do well?'

She lowered her head as if she'd been scolded and I worried that I'd expressed my frustration too harshly or been pulled into a punishing dialogue. This isn't uncommon in therapy – something about the way the young person perceives him or herself, or is perceived by someone else close to them, gets re-enacted in the transference. I didn't feel punishing towards Della – the opposite in fact – but I was aware that she might still perceive me as punishing and I decided to say so.

'I wonder if it feels like I'm telling you off, Della. I'm not. I'm just noticing that you often tell me you do things because of what other people want. I'm wondering what *you* want.'

'If I did what I want, I wouldn't be at school.'

'No?'

'No.'

'I wonder where you'd be?'

'Dead.'

'Dead?'

'Probably. Or getting wasted in a field. Being with Jimmy makes me less selfish.'

'I'm interested that you describe being dead and getting wasted in a field as selfish acts.'

'How would you describe them?'

'Let me think... I'd describe you being dead as very sad; you have a lot of life to live.'

'Maybe.'

'And I think the getting wasted part might be described as self-indulgent, perhaps, or self-absorbed, but I don't think I'd call it selfish.'

'My dad said I was selfish the last time I self-harmed. He saw my arm and said, "That's so fucking selfish".'

I know parents can be shocked when their child hurts themself; some react ragefully because they're angry or upset, but I thought we should unpick her father's response and what it meant for Della.

'What happened next, after he called you selfish?'

'He said that if I did it again, he'd cut his face in front of me.'

'Wow!'

'I know, right!'

'How did you respond to that?'
'I just stood there.'
'Until…?'
'Until he told me to have a shower and clean myself up.'

I was reminded of Della's story about the boy who had sex with her and then told her to clean herself up. I wondered (to myself) who it was (symbolically) that needed 'cleaning up' and who it was (symbolically) that was being attacked. It sounded as if Della's father had experienced his daughter's self-injury as an attack on *him*, but could it be that Della experienced it that way too? Freud had a similar line of inquiry in his paper, 'Whose Pain is it Really?' He suggested that often the most violent acts of self-hatred are less applicable to the patient himself but belong instead to someone whom 'the patient loves or has loved or should love' (Freud, 1917). Thought about in this way, Della's attack on her own body could represent a symbolic attack on someone else – her father, perhaps. Indeed, her father's threatened attack on his own body might also represent a symbolic attack on that of his daughter. It was complicated, but thought about symbolically and in the context of psychoanalytic theory, it seemed to me as if Della and her father had become enmeshed – as if each were carrying the projections of the other, and that Della's father had difficulty containing those of his daughter.

Bion spoke about the 'alpha function' of the parent, which involves using their own thoughts and feelings to hold, digest and make sense of those of the infant until they have the capacity to hold, digest and make sense of experiences for themselves (Bion, 1962). The good-enough parent acts as a container for the child's projections and provides what is arguably the primary task of parenting – and, I think, one of the primary tasks of psychotherapy too. Sometimes, the opposite happens – the container/contained relationship is reversed, and the parent's projections are forced into the child: 'Often it is the very adult who should have provided the function of containment, had he or she been fit to do so, who projects into the child' (G. Williams, 1997, p.103). Psychodynamic literature makes a distinction here between container and receptacle. A child cannot be a container for their parent, because they are but a child, but they can be used as a receptacle. I am not in the business of blaming parents for what is, after all, an unconscious process. But theories such as these can help me to frame my thinking and make sense of what might be going on. I was curious about Della's sense of herself as separate (or not) from her father and as separate (or not) from the men she had sex with.

Fucking around

A couple of weeks later, Della talked about meeting Kwame and spending an evening cuddled up with him, watching a movie. She said she would never cheat on Jimmy, but Kwame would always be special to her. He was an older – she didn't say how old – Nigerian boy she'd met 'years ago'. She'd thought she was in love with him once, but now they were just really good friends. Sometimes they 'messed around' together but he had a girlfriend and she had Jimmy. I asked if 'messed around' meant had sex and Della said, 'Yeah, kind of' and lowered her head. I said I wasn't judging her; she was entitled to have sex with whoever she wanted to, so long as it was consensual and safe, but I just wondered about the line between sexual and non-sexual relationships, which to me seemed blurry.

'It *is* blurry, you're right.'

'I wonder if you've thought about that before, Della?'

'No, not really.'

'I'm wondering if you ever have friendships with boys that aren't sexual.'

Della was quiet for several minutes and seemed to be working through a list in her mind of the boys she knew. Eventually she said, 'No, I don't think so.'

'Do you think that's unusual?'

'It depends on what you mean by unusual.'

I didn't want to seem punitive, so I asked, a bit clumsily perhaps, 'Well, do you think that's what it's like for other girls your age – that they don't hang out with boys without having sex?'

'Yeah, I think so.'

'So, do you think girls your age *could* hang out with boys without having sex?'

'No, I don't think so.'

'I wonder why…?'

'Because that's what they expect.'

'The boys?'

'Yeah, the boys.'

'I'm wondering about what the girls expect. Well, maybe not what they expect, what they *want*?'

Della shrugged, as if what girls wanted wasn't an issue that she'd given much consideration to. I asked, 'What do *you* want, Della?'

'I don't know.'

The next session, Della announced that she'd dumped Jimmy because he was getting too clingy. I wanted to congratulate her for taking control, but didn't because that related to my agenda, not hers. Instead, I wondered if she had been able to let him know the reason why she had split up with him.

She smiled and said, 'There's another reason, apart from the clinginess.'

'Oh…?'

'Kwame!'

I felt my heart sink. Ending the relationship hadn't been about taking control of how she wanted to be treated; it had been a replication of a familiar pattern of merging one sexual encounter with another, one relationship with the next. When I wondered what Kwame was like, if and how he was different to Jimmy, she described a rather exotic sounding, slightly out-of-reach, idealised boyfriend who had a job and his own flat and drove a car. He was 22. When girls tell me about their relationships with older men – Kwame was, after all, a man, not a boy, in the eyes of the law – alarm bells ring and I have to tread a fine balance between exploring what's going on and assessing risk, as I do with any other potential safeguarding issue. I began the exploration carefully.

'Kwame's quite a bit older than you. How did the two of you meet?'

'At a house party. He offered me a drink.'

'Go on…'

'We talked all night. And drank. And smoked some weed.'

'And afterwards…?'

'We met up again. And talked and drank and smoked some weed.'

'And had sex?'

'And had sex.'

'Drinking and smoking weed and having sex all sounds quite ordinary for someone your age, Della. But I'm wondering if you can put yourself in my position for a minute and think about what it's like for me to hear about you drinking and smoking weed and having sex with a man so much older than you are?'

'Oh, I think you'd like him. He's really nice!'

'It sounds like *you* might really like him, and *I* would really like it if you were with someone nice who treated you well. But still, I can't help being concerned about the age difference and what some people, your dad perhaps, might call "risky".'

'Shit, you're not gonna tell my dad, are you?'

'For now, no.'

'Thank God for that!'

'I'm glad you've told me about Kwame, so we can continue to think about this together and I can try to make sure you are keeping yourself safe. Can you agree to that, Della?' She agreed, verbally at least, to 'tell me everything'.

It's not uncommon for adolescents to tell me about risk, and for me to have to weigh up carefully what to do with what they tell me. I usually begin with an agreement that we'll both try to be honest with each other, such as the agreement I made with Della, and that if I believe they are potentially unsafe, I will have to think with them about that and we might have to include someone else in our thinking. There are no hard-and-fast rules, except the one about transparency.

First sex

The following session, Della arrived in a foul mood. On Saturday evening, she'd been having a shower when her phone rang. Seeing the name *Kwame* flash up on the screen, her dad answered it. She didn't know what the two men said to each other, but her dad burst into the bathroom and told her to 'get rid of that dirty, fucking black man' and when she tried to call Kwame later, she discovered that he'd blocked her number.

'How did that leave you feeling, Della?'

'Fucking fuming. How fucking dare he?'

'Your dad or Kwame?'

'Both! God, men are bastards!'

She didn't elaborate further but went on to tell me that Saturday had been a 'really bad day'. There was a party at her dad's flat and Della had invited her friend Billie. The two girls got 'really drunk' and 'really high'. She said they drank about four bottles of vodka between them, which seemed unlikely in reality, but I focused instead on the essence of the communication, which seemed to be that Della and her friend were off their heads with a bunch of older men and one of them was her dad.

'I'm wondering what it was about Saturday that was really bad, Della.'

'After the thing with my phone I was really pissed off and determined to get wasted.'

'At the party?'

'Yeah.'

'Go on…'

'One of my dad's friend's sons was there. His name's Kian. We used to go to school together, but they moved away at the end of Year 8 and I haven't seen him since.'

'Did you used to be friends with Kian?'

'Sort of. He took my virginity.'

'He took your virginity?'

'Yeah. Just before they left. It was the first time for both of us.'

'Just before they left…' I was doing the mental maths, 'So you were both…'

'We were both 13.'

'That's a really big deal.' She looked as if she felt punished by me, again, so I made myself clear. 'I mean first sex is a big deal and doing it at 13 is a big deal too.'

'I suppose.'

'I noticed that you said Kian *took* your virginity.'

'Yeah.'

'Took?'

'What do you mean?'

'Well, you could have said you *gave* your virginity, or you *lost* your virginity, but you said he *took* it.'

'Oh. Yeah.' She seemed curious about that too.

'Can you say more about what happened?'

'There's not much to tell. We were sort of going out and it just happened.'

'Can you remember what it was like?'

'A bit.'

'Are you able to say?'

'I didn't know what to do. I'd never done it before. We'd done blow jobs and stuff a couple of times…'

'Blow jobs and stuff?'

'Yeah, you know, I'd gone down on him.'

'Thank you for explaining, Della, I know what a blow job is!' It was feeling tense, and I needed to lighten the mood and help Della to feel comfortable again as we explored the uncomfortable themes

of first sex and whatever had happened on Saturday. It worked and I continued, 'How was that for you?'
'I didn't really like doing it.'
'But you did it with Kian a couple of times?'
'Yeah. He said he liked it.'
'And then you had sex for the first time?'
'Yeah.'
'Can you remember how you went from blow jobs to having sex?'
'He got on top of me and just, sort of, you know, put it in. I didn't know what he was doing at first.'
'And then?'
'And then I thought, shit, I'm having sex!'
'And what did it feel like to be having sex?'
'It didn't feel like anything.'

Della's depiction of first sex sounded clumsy, adolescent, not very well thought through but not so out of the ordinary either.

'And after that he moved away?'
'Yeah. And I didn't see him again. Until Saturday.'
'And then?'
'And then we did it again.'
'You and Kian had sex on Saturday?'
'Yeah.'
'Is that the really bad thing?'
'Yeah.'
'How so? You're not 13 anymore.'
'Well, you must think I fuck around with a different boy every week!'
'And it matters to you what I think of you?'
'Yeah, I suppose it does.'

It mattered to me that it mattered to Della; that she had a sense that what she did affected me, and that it affected me because I cared about her. I shared my sense that relationships were confusing for Della and that her sexual boundaries seemed muddled. I said that the first time we have sex sometimes sets up a pattern for the sex we'll go on to have later. She looked intrigued and so I continued. I said that, from what I'd heard about Della's first time, it sounded neither respectful nor fully consensual. It hadn't happened as part of a loving relationship, and it hadn't been very pleasurable for Della. The only person who seemed to have got their needs met was Kian, who left soon after it happened and wasn't seen again for three years. What Della wanted, or didn't want, hadn't come into it. And then came the eureka moment as Della exclaimed, 'And nothing's changed!'

'Not yet,' I agreed, 'But I think it will.'

Time for a change

Things did change for Della, both in therapy and in the real world. I noticed that in sessions we felt more connected, she was more engaged in thinking and reflecting, rather than recounting endless tales of her 'fuck-ups'. In one session, during a comfortable silence of several minutes, I observed Della picking at a tiny hole in her tights, which soon became a long ladder that ran all the way down her leg from her thigh to her ankle. She realised what she'd done, looked up and made eye contact with me.

I met her gaze and said, 'Oh.'

'I'm a mess.'

'Your tights certainly are.'

'And my shoes.' She angled her foot to show me that the sole was loose.

'Yes, and your shoes.'

'It's not just that though, look at the state of me.'

'I'm looking at you, Della. What do you suppose I see?'

'An ugly fuck-up.'

'I don't see an ugly fuck-up at all. I see a bright, funny, attractive young woman, doing her best to do better.'

'You're paid to say that!'

'I'm paid to be honest.'

'Touché!'

'Joking aside, that *is* what I see, and I *am* being honest. I think you've been honest with me, and you deserve the same in return.'

'I have. And thanks.' She smiled.

'My sense is that you've rubbished yourself, sometimes by cutting, sometimes by drinking and sometimes by having sex with boys who treat you like rubbish.'

'I suppose.'

'It's become a bit of a self-fulfilling prophecy. Do you know what I mean by that?'

'Yeah. I think I'm rubbish, so people treat me like I'm rubbish.'

'Yes, maybe. But I also think that thinking of yourself as rubbish must have come from somewhere in the first place. You must have got that idea of yourself from the way you felt you were being treated.'

'My mum always said I was a clingy baby.'

'You think your view of yourself might come from when you were a baby?'

'Maybe.'

'I think so too. What do you think about that clingy baby?'

'It's terrifying!'

'Terrifying?'

'Yeah. To be so needy and so dependent on someone else.'

'That's what babies are, though, Della, dependent on their parents to meet their needs. Maybe it's the idea that those needs might not be met that's terrifying?'

I noticed that Della had watery eyes, something she hadn't let me see before. She was in touch with some difficult feelings that felt raw and real and sad.

'I think I had to learn not to depend on my mum and dad because of Kiki. The first time she went into hospital I was only seven and I had to just get on with it.'

'Get on with it?'

'Yeah.'

'With what?'

'With my life. I started smoking.'

'At seven?'

'Yeah, about that age. And before long I was drinking.'

'Do you think you were trying to be a grown up?'

'Yeah, I suppose I was.'

'But you weren't a grown up, Della, you were a little girl and you needed to be looked after, like your sister.'

'I know. I think that's why I started going with boys.'

'To feel looked after?'

'Yeah.'

'That makes sense. You didn't feel noticed at home, so you got people to notice you elsewhere. And then I suppose your parents noticed you even less because you weren't around so much and you gave off the impression that you could look after yourself, that you didn't need to depend on them or be a "clingy baby" any more.'

'So, it's my sister's fault?' she said, only half jokingly.

'I don't think it's about finding fault; it's about understanding how you became you. Your sister isn't to blame for her mental illness, your parents aren't to blame for being so overwhelmed by looking after her that you sometimes had to look after yourself, and you're not to blame for going off the rails a bit.'

'That's an understatement!'

'Is it? What would you call it?'

'I fucked up.'

'Whose words are those, Della? Who thinks you've fucked up?'

'My dad.'

I thought again about the father/daughter relationship and my hypothesis about the reversal of the container/contained relationship.

'Maybe he feels like he fucked up too. Maybe there's a part of him that feels responsible for letting you down. I'm not making excuses; I'm just saying there's a different perspective we could consider here.'

'I hadn't thought about that. Maybe the reason he's always prodding and poking is because he doesn't want me to end up like Kiki.'

'In hospital?'

'Yeah.'

'Maybe.'

'I feel bad now.'

'Maybe he does too, but there's no need. Maybe now you're spending more time together, you can begin to see each other's perspectives a bit more clearly.'

'We went out for a walk the other day.'

'You and your dad?'

'Yeah.'

'How was that?'

'Nice. We walked round the park and there was this balloon shaped like a heart stuck up a tree.'

'Yeah…' I smiled at the image. 'What did you make of that?'

'I thought it was quite symbolic. Love sometimes gets stuck!'

'Absolutely! My sense is that you were a bit like that balloon when I met you.'

'Yeah, I needed rescuing.'

'Mmm, I don't think you needed rescuing. I think maybe you were feeling a bit deflated, like your bubble had been burst and you were stuck.'

She smiled, and I did too, and we both recognised that things had changed and that she was ready to begin the process of ending therapy. Della had come to therapy feeling clumsy and awkward, unsure how to recognise or communicate her own needs, let alone how to ensure they were met. She had internalised a sense of herself as unremarkable and unworthy – the 'bad' sister whose share of her parents' attention was felt to be taken by the 'mad' sister. She tried her best to prove to me that she was a useless fuck-up who wasn't worth noticing or caring about. But I did notice her, and I did care.

I thought about the behaviour Della told me about in the context of her family experiences. The acting out, the risky and sexually promiscuous behaviour, often with older boys and young men, seemed to be communicating her unmet needs – *notice me, care about me, love me* – as risky or unhealthy behaviour often does. I didn't judge the behaviour or condone it. I let Della know when I was concerned, and I encouraged her to exert her right to choose what happened to her and make sense of why this had been so hard for her to do in the past. For reasons that were beyond the scope of Della's therapy, but almost certainly included the demands of caring for their older, mentally unwell daughter, Della's parents had not been able to hold, digest and make sense of their younger child. I think that therapy provided this 'alpha function' (Bion, 1962), and the experience of a relationship in which Della was cared about and felt contained. My sense was that she began to internalise those positive aspects of the therapeutic relationship and hold onto a sense of renewed self-worth.

As we navigated our ending period, Della was spending more time with her dad, going out for walks and chatting about 'normal stuff'. She was single, drinking and smoking less and attending school regularly. To quote Della, she had decided to 'quit fucking around'.

4

In transition

Lane is confused – about their gender, their sexuality, about everything. Can psychotherapy help them to make sense of their adolescent thoughts and feelings so they can become their authentic self?

. . . .

Melanie was referred to me for psychotherapy by her GP. He wrote that she was displaying symptoms of anxiety and depression, including self-harming behaviour. Melanie had not attended school for more than a year. She had been assigned a home tutor but found it difficult to engage, with them and with learning. The GP stated that Melanie spent all day at home in her bedroom, sitting in the dark, and that he and her family were concerned about her deteriorating mental health. I was told that Melanie lived with her maternal grandmother but had a good relationship with her mother.

I wrote to the family address, inviting Melanie to attend for an initial consultation, along with a parent or alternative adult. I explained that this would be an opportunity for me to learn more about the current concerns and family background, as well as a chance for Melanie to meet me and decide if she would like to have some individual psychotherapy sessions with me. Melanie attended with her mother, Gill. She was sturdily built and tall for her age. Her blond hair was dyed green and cut short and was mostly hidden under a black beanie hat that was pulled down over her eyebrows. She wore no make-up. Her skin looked sallow, and her eyes were bloodshot, as if she had been crying or had a late night, or maybe both. Melanie's clothes were nondescript and shapeless and didn't seem to fit her. In contrast to many of the adolescent girls I meet, Melanie seemed to have dressed simply to clothe her body, without regard for how she looked.

These observations are not meant to sound disrespectful. It's important for me to acknowledge what I notice about a young person when I meet them for the first time, and my thoughts about those observations, because they form the beginnings of my clinical formulations and hypotheses. My first thoughts about Melanie were that she didn't seem to care much about or for herself and that the way that she presented didn't make sense to me.

I made my introductions and invited Melanie to tell me why she had come to see me. She looked tearful and remained silent, before mumbling, almost inaudibly, 'Mum can say.' I asked Gill if she could help by explaining what was worrying her. She said, 'Melanie's dropped out of school. She can't cope.'

'She can't cope…?' I repeated, encouraging her to continue.

'No. With the bullying.'

'I'm sorry to hear you've been bullied.' I addressed Melanie directly. 'And so you left?'

She nodded and Gill continued, 'She won't get her exams and won't be able to go to college.'

'That's a real shame. And you must be worried about what kind of future Melanie will have, with no qualifications.'

I was interested in Melanie's present, as well as her future, and I wondered aloud what she did all day.

'She sleeps.' Gill stated. 'She's up all night and in bed all day.'

I registered this topsy-turvy, upside-down kind of existence and continued my exploration of Melanie's home life. When I enquired who lived at home, Gill raised her eyebrows in an *it's complicated* kind of way. I established that Melanie had a younger sister called Paige, who lived permanently at home with mum, and an older sister called Clare, who came and went. Melanie had 'sort of' moved out to live with her nan because she didn't get on with Clare's boyfriend, who often stayed at the house, but he and Clare had currently broken up and so Melanie was back at home. It certainly did sound complicated, and I was struck by the instability of Melanie's life – all the comings and goings and the blurred lines about who lived where and when, as well as the distortions I had already noted between night and day.

Gill went on to describe further worries about Melanie. I heard that she had no routine in terms of sleeping or eating and that she seldom left the house. Gill said that Melanie spent all her time on the computer, and when I glanced at Melanie, she nodded her agreement. When I asked what she did, she said she liked to play fantasy games and she also liked to create computer-generated art. I heard that she had been good at art at school and had hoped to study it at college, 'until all this'. Gill was aware of some previous self-injury but didn't think Melanie was harming herself now. I looked across at Melanie again and detected a look that urged me not to go there, so I didn't request any elaboration, but stored this away for future exploration. When I enquired about social contact, Melanie told me that she had friends who visited her at home. She named a few in particular and described them as people she enjoyed hanging out with. She said she rarely went out of the house with them, because she was too anxious and had experienced panic attacks in the past when she was away from home. I wondered to myself what kind of friends these might be, and what benefits they might gain from their (mostly nocturnal) visits to Melanie's house.

I asked, 'I wonder if you have any idea about what might be causing you to panic and experience low moods?'

'Everyone stares at me.'

'You think everyone stares at you?'

'I don't think it, I know it. They think I'm a freak.'

'Gosh, that's quite a statement. Why would they think you're a freak?'

'Because I am.'

'*You* think you're a freak?'

'Yes.'

'That sounds like a harsh thought to have about yourself.'

'What do you mean?'

'It doesn't sound very kind.'

'I suppose so.'

'You might not be able to answer this question, but I'm wondering why you think of yourself that way?'

'Because I'm trans.'

I checked I'd understood by asking, 'You identify as transgender?'

'Yes.'

'And you think that makes you a freak?'

'Yes.'

'Freak seems like a really negative term, and I'm sorry you have assigned that label to yourself, but I can understand why you, and others, might be struggling to understand why you feel – I don't know – different.'

Melanie looked at me, as if interested, but didn't speak. I wasn't sure I'd got it right and so I clarified my statement by thinking aloud.

'By "different" I think I mean different perhaps to how you once felt, and different to some of your peers. And I'm also acknowledging that there might be a difference between how you feel on the inside and how you are on the outside. Am I on the right lines?'

'Absolutely. All of that.'

'Good. I wanted to check. Sometimes words mean different things to different people. Talking about different, your mum introduced you to me as Melanie, is that the name you prefer?

'No. I hate it.'

'She prefers "Lane",' Gill stated, and I clocked the use of the pronoun 'she'.

'Lane.' I said the name aloud. 'Would you prefer me to use that name?'

'Yes, please.'

'And which pronouns?'

'I use they/them.'

'Okay. I'll use those too.'

[A side note here: I strive to meet all young people where they're at with affirmation and give them a space to explore all aspects of themselves, including the hidden or split-off parts. What it means to be young, trans, non-binary or questioning is all too often defined by society, culture, parents, patriarchy or policy, rather than by young, trans, non-binary or questioning people themselves. For resources to support young trans, gender variant and gender questioning people aged 8–30, I frequently point people towards the all-inclusive charity Gendered Intelligence.[1] For reliable information about trans and non-binary people's legal rights, including rights to healthcare and recognition, I recommend TransActual,[2] a charity committed to overcoming transphobia and misinformation. Because we all have the capacity to be allies, whatever our gender or sexuality.]

I noticed that Gill had started to cry. She said she was aware of how Lane felt and that the family was supportive. Despite her words of encouragement, I noted that she had referred to Lane as her daughter and misgendered her by using the pronoun 'she'. A name is often a

---

1. https://genderedintelligence.co.uk/
2. www.transactual.org.uk/

signifier of gender. Some names are unisex, of course – but most give an indication as to whether a person is male or female. When someone changes their name, it can be a declaration that they have changed or denounced the gender assigned to them at birth. For transgender people, choosing a new name can be an act of self-definition and a rite of passage (Holleb, 2019). It can be empowering. It says, 'This is me; this is who I am and how I want to be identified.' But it can also be fraught with difficulty and tension, depending on how those around the individual react. I took Gill's use of 'Melanie', 'daughter' and 'she/her' pronouns as a potential signifier of ambivalence.

I realised that we had reached what was perhaps at the core of Lane's issues, and also that we were out of time for our first session. I turned to Lane and said that it was clear to me that they were struggling to manage some difficult feelings, and that perhaps it might be helpful to have someone outside of the family to explore this with. Lane accepted my offer of six individual psychotherapy sessions rather more eagerly than I had anticipated. It seemed they were ready.

Ambivalence

Lane arrived 20 minutes late for their first individual session, brought by Gill, who waited outside in the car. I had waited for Lane in my therapy room and reflected on our initial meeting. As the time ticked by, I wondered if they would come at all. I was aware of my growing anxiety about what might be keeping Lane from their appointment. I wondered if they had changed their mind, or if they had set off and had a panic attack, or if they had just not managed to get out of bed. I was relieved when Lane finally arrived and told them I was pleased to see them. Lane didn't refer to the fact that they were late, and I didn't ask for an explanation. Instead, I stated that we would have 'until 10 to', motioning towards the clock on the wall, which now showed 20 past. It was important for me to hold the boundaries, which were already being tested. Because I had heard so much about Lane's blurred and un-boundaried lifestyle at the initial consultation, it was no surprise to me that these themes were being played out in therapy from the start. Themes and patterns from the 'real world' often get replicated in therapy and it's important to acknowledge them. In Freudian terms, this is the 'repetition compulsion' – the tendency to unconsciously act out something from the past in the here and now (Freud, 1920).

I acknowledged that Lane's mum had done most of the talking the first time we met and said it would be good to hear more about Lane from Lane themself. I remembered (to myself) that they had identified as trans, and wondered (to myself) whether this represented the first steps of our therapeutic journey. Sometimes, explorations of gender begin more vaguely and work towards a label; other times, they begin with the label and work outwards (Roche, 2020). I didn't verbalise my thoughts because where we began was up to Lane. They told me they wanted to be male and had left school because no one could accept that. They said everyone thought they were a freak. I wondered what Lane thought about themself, and they started to cry. I acknowledged how hard it seemed for Lane to tell me about their experiences and encouraged them to take their time, but to tell me what they could about their feelings.

'I've felt the same since Year 7.'

'The same?'

'The same as I do now.'

'Can you help me to understand what that feeling feels like?'

'Like I am a boy.'

'And you first became aware of that in Year 7, the year you started secondary school?'

'Yes.'

In my experience of working with young people, the transition to secondary school, accompanied by the onset of puberty, is often the time when feelings about gender and sexuality come to the fore. Young people start to question, or question more vociferously, who they are, what they feel and who they are and aren't attracted to.

I noticed that Lane had said both that they *wanted* to be male and that they *felt like* they were a boy – statements that differ subtlety, but significantly. 'I want to be…' suggests a desire to be something you're not, while 'I am…' suggests the opposite. Perhaps this illustrated something of the fluidity of Lane's thought processes about their gender development, as well as the fluidity of gender itself – both very ordinary and common processes, particularly during adolescence. In the introduction to her brilliant book *Gender Explorers*, Juno Roche states that children question and explore their gender in order to lead happy, functional and aspirational lives (Roche, 2020). It was painfully evident that Lane was neither happy nor functioning, and I attempted to build some context around their experience of gender identity.

'I'm wondering what life in Year 7 was like for you?'
'Hard.'
'How so?'
'We'd just moved.'
'Moved house?'
'Yes. To be nearer my nan.'
'The one you sometimes stay with?'
'Yes.'
'Where were you before that?'
'We'd lived in the same place since before I was born.'

Lane named a town a couple of hours' drive away and I acknowledged that the move must have been experienced as a big upheaval. I learnt that Nan was divorced, but had a male friend, and that Lane had never known their maternal grandfather. The family script described him as a violent man who had had no relationship with his daughter, Lane's mother. Lane's description of their own father depicted a weak and occasionally aggressive man, who left their mother when Lane was an infant. He was also father to Lane's younger sister Paige, and had been in and out of their lives, causing considerable disruption to family life. Lane had decided, from about the age of nine, that they didn't want anything to do with him. He continued irregular contact with Paige and, according to Lane, attempted to maintain control over Gill. Lane's older sister Clare had a different father, and had maintained an intermittent relationship with him. All too quickly our session was over. I had been struck by the story of family instability, the erratic relationships and the capricious fathers who came and went. I wondered how this had influenced Lane's sense of self, identity and gender, and their relationship with male role models.

The developing body

When we met again, Lane arrived early and said they had found it helpful to talk to me in the previous session. In an effort to ascertain whether they were just being polite, I asked, 'I wonder what was helpful in particular.'

'I'm not sure.'

'Has anything stayed with you from our previous session?'

'We talked about my family,' Lane said, in a rather non-committal way.

'I've been remembering that too,' I said, to join with Lane and let them know I'd kept them in mind. 'Was there anything that stood out for you in what we talked about?'

'I'm not sure.'

It was early days in the therapy, and this way of thinking wasn't yet familiar to Lane, so I shared what had stayed with me.

'I've been thinking that the way you described the men in your family made them sound pretty unreliable.'

They raised their eyebrows in the same *it's complicated* way I had noticed from their mother during the initial consultation.

'I wonder if there are any other male role models in your life who are different to your dad, or your sister's dad or your grandad?'

'My uncle.'

'Can you tell me about him?'

'He's my mum's brother. We get on really well.'

'That's good to hear. Do you spend much time together?'

'Yes. He knows about me, and he lets me have some of his clothes.'

'He knows you're transgender?'

'Yes.'

'And he accepts you for who you are?'

'Yes.'

I realised then that Lane was dressed in their uncle's hand-me-downs, which explained why they were loose and shapeless and didn't fit them properly. Or rather, Lane didn't seem to fit the clothes properly, because they were bought to fit a different man, rather than them. This made some sense of my feeling that Lane wasn't presenting as themself. I wondered too what it might symbolise about Lane's sense of 'not fitting' – in the clothes, in the family or in their own female body. I was reminded of a book by Jamie Windust. Jamie is a writer, editor, model and public speaker who advocates for the rights of LGBTQA+ people and calls out misogynistic, homophobic and transphobic behaviour. Their book *In Their Shoes* (Windust, 2021) is both an exploration and a navigation of their queer life – their trials and tribulations and, inevitably (they're a model), their clothes and shoes. I wanted to explore what it was like to be in Lane's clothes and shoes.

'Can you tell me about the clothes?'

'I like men's clothes because they are more comfortable.'

'More comfortable how?'

'They're dark and baggy and… I'm not sure… the opposite of feminine, I suppose.'

'So, they feel more comfortable to wear?'

'Yes.'

'And I wonder if *you* feel more comfortable while you're wearing them? More comfortable inside, I mean.'

'Yes. I feel male and I want other people to see me as male, so I wear male clothes.'

This made sense, in theory, but in reality there was something missing; Lane *didn't* seem comfortable. I became aware of my own attire – dress, boots, jewellery – distinctly feminine clothes that I felt comfortable in. I wondered to myself what my appearance was communicating to Lane: certainly, that I was female; possibly, that I was different to them, and perhaps that I wouldn't understand. I didn't understand, not yet, and so I encouraged them to tell me more about what it was like for Lane to be Lane.

Lane described the daily ritual of binding their large breasts with bandages in an attempt to flatten them. Over the bandages they wore at least two tight-fitting Lycra vests, followed by a t-shirt and then a looser sweatshirt or jumper as a final, outer layer. I felt terribly sad that biology had given Lane the body shape they had, and how difficult it must be for them to conceal it. As if reading my thoughts, Lane said they wished their breasts were smaller, and I felt self-conscious once more, as I'm certain they did too. So much was being communicated between us through our bodies, both physically and symbolically. I decided to open up the exploration and enquired as to when their body had started to develop and if they could recall what that was like.

'These grew overnight,' Lane said, indicating their chest.

'Overnight? Gosh! Do you remember when that was?'

'When I started Year 7.'

'So, you were about 11?'

'Yeah… and I got my period that same week.'

'Your first period?'

'Yeah.'

'That's a lot to get used to all at once.'

'It was, yeah.'

'And I remember you telling me that was when you moved house?'

'Oh yes, it was.'

'I'm wondering how ready you were for those changes?'
'What do you mean?'
'Well, I think I mean practically ready for the changes in your body. Did you have the stuff you needed? Sanitary stuff, a bra?'
'I had pads.'
'From your mum?'
'From Clare.'
'Your sister?'
'Yeah.'
'Had she explained to you what they were for and how to use them?'
'No. No one told me anything about periods or anything, really. Clare just threw a pack of pads onto my bed one day and told me I'd probably need them soon. I think I was about eight or nine. I didn't really know what they were for.'
'That sounds confusing.'
Lane shrugged.

I was struck, as I often am when speaking with young people, by Lane's lack of preparedness for puberty. Sex education at school is frequently sparse and often belated, while sex education at home is often delivered awkwardly, or not at all. I'd asked Lane about how practically ready they were for the inevitable changes their body would go through, but linked to my question about practical readiness was a curiosity about emotional preparedness. When practical information and resources, such as bras and feminine hygiene products, are presented in a careful and timely way, this can also help young people to be more emotionally ready for puberty. It was apparent that Lane had been neither practically nor emotionally prepared for the changes their body would go through.

Self-loathing

I noted too the timing of their 'overnight' development, which coincided with Lane's transition to secondary school and the family moving home. This was the time they first became aware of their physiologically female sexual development and rejected it. It was a lot to deal with, but I had a sense that there might be something else, some other trigger for the self-loathing. It was important to go at the pace set by Lane, and I decided to explore further their choice of clothes, as it was something we'd already begun to think about together.

It was evident that the baggy outer garments were disguising multiple layers of physical as well as emotional pain. When I commented on how uncomfortable the binding sounded, Lane told me that the bandages cut into their skin and sometimes they rubbed and caused bleeding.

'That sounds so painful.'

'It is, yeah, but I have to do it.'

'You *have* to do it.'

'Yeah.'

'Tell me about that...'

'What do you mean?'

'Well, when you say you *have* to do something, it's sounds almost like, I don't know, almost like a compulsion. Like you're compelled to bind your breasts.'

Lane thought for a moment and then replied, 'I suppose it is a compulsion, in a way, because it's the only thing I feel like I have to do every single day.'

'Every day, no matter what you're doing?'

'Yeah, even if I'm not going out, or if no one's coming over.'

'So, it's something you do for you, not for other people?'

'It is, yeah.'

'There's nothing else you do every day, just for yourself?'

'Like what?'

'I'm not sure... maybe showering... washing your hair... choosing what to wear?'

Lane told me that they hated showering or taking a bath because they couldn't bear to touch themself 'from the neck down'. They said that sometimes the wounds from binding became infected, but they couldn't touch or clean them because they couldn't bear to look. I wondered how they managed their periods and they said they were repulsive. They couldn't bear to see the blood coming out of them and so they didn't bathe or shower at all during menstruation. The way that Lane described their infected, self-inflicted wounds and their lack of sanitary hygiene did indeed sound repulsive. I felt desperately unhappy that Lane's body was not being looked after or nurtured and that it had instead become a source of disgust.

'That makes me feel sad for your body, Lane.'

They looked at me expectantly and I continued, 'It's like how you're treating your body is the opposite of self-care. In fact, I'm thinking of

it, in a way, as a kind of self-harm.'
   'I suppose.'
   'Does that make sense to you, even if you don't see it that way?'
   'Sort of.'
   'What I'm hearing you say is that sometimes you don't take care of your body by washing or managing your period or treating your wounds when they get infected.'
   Lane looked upset.
   'You're not being kind to your body.'
   'No.'
   'I'm wondering if you ever hurt yourself in other ways, maybe more deliberate ways?'
   'Sometimes.'
   'Are you able to tell me about that?'
   'Sometimes I use cigarettes.'
   'Cigarettes?'
   'Yeah.'
   'To burn yourself?'
   'Yeah, here.' Lane pointed to their chest. 'And sometimes I cut here and here.' They pointed to their abdomen and inner thighs.
   I sensed an enormous amount of self-loathing, which Lane was acting out in violent acts against their own body. The room was filled with a heavy sadness that lingered long after they had left.

Self-injury

When young people share with me acts of intentional self-injury, I'm faced with an ethical dilemma. I have a duty of care to assess the immediate risk and to act in a way that safeguards the young person. Adolescent psychotherapists may be bound by the safeguarding policies of the organisation that employs them. This can make ethical decision-making more straightforward, because there is clear guidance that says, 'If this happens, you must do that.' It can also be frustrating, if the individual therapist doesn't agree with the organisational policies. Working in private practice, I contract with each young person in the first session. I tell them that what we do and say in therapy is private, with a couple of exceptions. I explain that I might think over the content and process of their therapy with my supervisor, so that, if there's a difficult dilemma, I have help to consider the options. As well as being transparent, I think this also models the fact that I'm not sitting here with all the answers; I'm human and fallible and benefit from support too.

This leads nicely onto *when* additional support might be called upon. I tell young people that, if I'm concerned about their immediate safety, I will need to check that out with them in more detail. Sometimes, I might ask if it's okay to include a parent or carer in our thinking, in order to keep them safe, and sometimes I might need to take it to supervision. The times when I need to over-ride their wishes and include parents or carers in thinking about their child's self-injury are exceptionally rare and, because I work in private practice, I never have to share or report incidents with anyone else either. I am a firm believer in the right to confidentiality, in and out of the therapy room, including the right to protection against parental intrusion. As Melanie Klein stated, the child or young person deserves the same right to confidentiality as the adult (Klein, 1932).

Research posits a wide range of risk factors for self-injury in adolescents, including age, gender, ethnicity, mental and physical health and family circumstances. The act itself has been described, somewhat derogatorily, as attention seeking or a cry for help. Each of these terms, if considered benignly, can be seen as describing a form of communication. Attention-seeking behaviour says, 'Notice me'; a cry for help says, 'Listen to me'. An alternative way of understanding self-injury is as a 'cry of pain' (J. Williams, 1997). This model sees self-injury as a reaction to circumstances in which the individual feels trapped, with no means of escape or rescue. This way of thinking seemed to me to make sense of Lane's sense of being trapped, not only in their own 'repulsive' body, as they saw it, but also in their own confused mind. The body was being attacked, ritually and compulsively, through over-zealous binding and lack of self-care, as well as more deliberately through burning and cutting. For Lane, self-injury had become a way of coping with their confusing thoughts and emotions, which I was beginning to understand as possible gender dysphoria – a feeling of incongruence related to the gender assigned at birth (Holleb, 2019).

So, what to do about Lane's self-injury and how could I help? There are a number of viable options that *can* be effective for *some* people. These include avoidance or distraction – in other words, encouraging them to do something else instead of injuring themselves; deterrence – in other words, suggesting they delay self-injury until later; and minimisation – asking them not to do it so severely. To suggest any of these strategies to Lane would have felt directive, dismissive of the reasons behind the self-injury and, to a lesser extent, punitive. I didn't want to come across in any of those ways. I respected their right to use whatever coping mechanisms they relied upon. I also trusted in the process of psychotherapy (enough) and in our therapeutic relationship (enough) to know that talking would help and that understanding the meaning behind the self-injury was likely to alleviate the need to do it (Fox & Hawton, 2004).

Projection

Lane missed their next appointment. I didn't hear from them or their mother and I worried that I might have pushed Lane too much, and too soon, in the previous session. This is an anxiety I often experience when a client doesn't come back in the early days of therapy. I ask myself what I might have done wrong, whether I've been too intrusive, or the opposite – not seemed interested enough. When I reflected on the previous session, I had a sense of it as very raw, just as Lane's wounds must have been raw. Perhaps they needed more time to heal before they came back. When clients don't attend, I have an additional dilemma about whether or not to make contact and, if so, whether the contact should be directed towards the young person themself or their parent. In this instance, I decided not to contact Lane or their family at all, but to respect their decision not to attend their session.

When Lane didn't attend for a second consecutive week, I grew more concerned. I waited in my therapy room, reflecting on the previous weeks, and towards the end of the session time I decided to telephone the family. Gill told me that Lane had been enthusiastic about therapy and said that they experienced the first couple of sessions as 'really helpful'. They didn't come last week because they weren't feeling well, and today, Gill had been busy and so Lane was supposed to make their own way to their appointment but hadn't. Gill asked me to 'give her another chance' and 'not give her slot to someone else because she really needs it'. I asked Gill to give a message to Lane that I'd been thinking about them and looked forward to seeing them next week.

The conversation with Gill was interesting. I registered her continued use of 'her' and 'she'. I wondered what Lane's not feeling well the previous week might have been about – was it a physical or an emotional unwellness? I wondered why Gill hadn't let me know at the time. She had made a decision, consciously or not, to leave me waiting and wondering, in a state of not-knowing – an uncomfortable position to be in. I wondered if this was a projection onto me of her own uncomfortable feelings.

Projection can be thought about as a way of disowning difficult feelings and giving them to someone else to feel instead. It is one of a number of defence mechanisms, first posited by Sigmund Freud and later developed by his daughter Anna, that are unconsciously used to protect a person from uncomfortable or unacceptable thoughts or feelings. Psychodynamic theory suggests five main psychological defence mechanisms (Freud, 1937): repression defends the conscious mind by forcing from conscious awareness thoughts that are difficult to know, feel or be aware of; regression involves retreating mentally, emotionally and/or physically to an earlier stage of development where there was less anxiety – usually a return to a childlike or infantile state; reaction formation involves doing the exact opposite of what is desired but deemed unacceptable, often in an over-the-top or excessive way, and sublimation is a defence that transforms undesirable or unacceptable emotions or instincts into healthy, socially acceptable behaviours.

The projections from our clients (and their families) can give us clues about how they are feeling when they are unaware of those thoughts, or unable or unwilling to tell us about them in words. As well as being aware of the not-knowing position I had been pulled into sharing with Gill, I also wondered if the non-attendance symbolised ambivalence about psychotherapy and, if so, whether that ambivalence belonged to Gill or to Lane. In our brief telephone conversation, Gill had made a desperate sounding plea about her child's need for therapy and about me giving them another chance. I thought this was a strange request to ask of a therapist – *'Give her another chance'* – as if Gill felt that I had been let down in some way. It sounded like the kind of thing an unfaithful partner might say (or perhaps a disloyal parent?) – *'Give me another chance'*, with the insinuation, *'I promise I'll do better next time.'* I wondered what this might be communicating about disloyalty within the family system: did Gill feel disloyal to Lane perhaps, because of her own ambivalence about their gender identification? I could only hypothesise, but I decided to hold in mind that the idea of disloyalty had now been projected into the therapeutic sphere as an additional theme for consideration.

'Fine'

Lane arrived for their next session 10 minutes late. I said I was pleased to see them and that we had until 10 to the hour. They asked if they were late, and I reminded them that their sessions were at 11 o'clock until 11.50. They looked at the clock as if they were registering this for the first time. It was certainly the first time they had acknowledged being late, illustrating a new awareness of the boundaries of the sessions. I acknowledged that we hadn't seen each other for a few weeks and I said I'd been wondering how they'd been. Lane said 'fine' – a response I often hear from adolescents, but always check out further. There was a time when young people used FINE as an acronym that meant 'fucked up, insecure and neurotic'. In my experience, fine doesn't often mean fine.

'And what's *fine* been like for you this week?' I asked with a smile.

'Shit.'

'I'm sorry to hear that, Lane. What would you like me to know about your shit week?'

'I've cried a lot and not really slept very much. And I've self-harmed.'

'I'm sorry to hear that too.'

'I'm really tired.'

'Yes, it does sound exhausting. Managing painful emotion can use up a lot of energy, and if you aren't getting much sleep, you'll have no reserves. No wonder you're tired.'

'Yeah, I know. I usually stay in bed until about four.'

'Four in the afternoon?'

'Yeah.' Lane yawned, highlighting just how exhausted they wanted me to know they were.

'And today you got up early to come here. I'm impressed.'

I *was* impressed, and I think it's important to acknowledge the effort it takes some young people just to get up, get dressed and get out of the house, and how depleting it can be to have shit week after shit week. I also noticed that Lane had made a point of telling me they usually stayed in bed until four in the afternoon, and yet here they were, meeting me, at 11 in the morning. Were they letting me know the sessions were important to them, worth getting up for perhaps? I hoped so. Lane *had* turned up, during their usual sleeping hours, and seemed ready to engage.

I remembered aloud that they had told me before that they usually stayed up most of the night and slept during the day. I wondered if they could tell me more about that.

'I like the night better.'

'Go on...'

'I like the dark and the quiet.'

'Yes...'

'And I like that I'm doing something different to what everyone else is doing.'

'I'm curious about that, about the sense of doing something different, is that something that's important to you, the difference?'

'Well, I *am* different. I don't know anyone else like me!'

'Can you say more?'

'Anyone who is like I am. Anyone who is, you know.' They trailed off as if it was too difficult to say the words.

I checked I had understood, 'Do you mean anyone who feels like they don't fit in their body?'

Lane nodded, so I named explicitly what I thought we were referring to, 'Anyone who is transgender?' Again, Lane nodded, but this time they looked me right in the eye.

'It seems painful for you to have this sense of being different. It must be hard to carry the feeling around with you, that no one is like you or understands you.'

I could see that Lane was really hooked into me, attentive to what I was going to say next, so I decided to carry on thinking aloud.

'I've been thinking about your topsy-turvy way of life, sleeping in the day and being awake at night when it's quiet and dark. Some people describe the quiet of the night as a frightening time, but for you, the opposite seems to be true, it's less frightening than the daytime.'

Lane nodded and so I continued some more.

'For you, there seems to be something about the dark and the quiet and the solitude that you like. You can't be judged if there's no one around to judge you. You can't be ridiculed if everyone else is asleep. You can be whoever you are.'

I remembered that Lane had mentioned online chat forums where they took up various gender and sexual identities. In this way they had been able to explore and experiment in relative safety. If they received a negative comment or a harsh response, they could delete it, or present differently, or switch off their laptop. Lane also told me that, as well as pretending to be other people online, they could be themself. When I wondered who that was, they whispered 'trans'.

Over time, Lane began to talk more openly to me about sex. They said they hadn't experienced penetrative sex, although they had experimented with masturbation and oral sex with same-aged peers, both male and female. They said they identified as 'pan'. As with 'fine', I always check out with young people the meaning of their words, even if I think I understand, and especially when they use jargon or abbreviations. As with 'fine', the term 'pan' can mean different things to different people and the sense I make of their response differs too.

'You identify as pan. I'm wondering what that means, for you?'

'You don't know what pan means?'

'I know what it means to me, but I'm interested to know what it means for you.'

'It means I'm attracted to people of any gender or sexuality.'

This felt like a stock answer. I wondered if Lane's identification as 'pan' was ambiguous, and whether it illustrated confusion rather than certainty, which is quite ordinary, of course, for someone of 16. I'd noticed their identification as 'pan' rather than pan-*sexual* and 'trans' rather than trans-*gender*, again quite common and ordinary abbreviations, but I didn't want to dismiss the potential significance of what hadn't been named – sex and gender. I contemplated how difficult it must be for a young person struggling with their sense of gender identity, which is assumed to be fixed, to make sense of their sexuality, which is assumed to be related, and how they might struggle to put that into words.

The terms used to describe and define gender and sexual identity can be confusing. Pansexual is often used interchangeably with bisexual to mean, as Lane had stated, attraction regardless of gender. However, some individuals choose pansexual over bisexual, arguing that the latter reduces sexuality to two (bi) identities: heterosexual and homosexual. Others argue that both terms, but especially bisexual, are transphobic, because they implicitly suggest attraction to the 'same and opposite genders' (Holleb, 2019). Other, more expansive, terms include polysexual and omnisexual, which describe attraction to *multiple* genders, including transgender. It's important to notice and respect the labels that each individual chooses to describe themselves, their experiences and their preferences, and to explore what those labels mean to them. I've already mentioned that sex education is frequently sparse, belated, and delivered awkwardly. Thankfully, there is a growing number of contemporary, thorough, honest resources that discuss sex and gender in way that feels inclusive for people born with a penis or a vulva, whatever their sexual or gender orientation. For younger children, I commend *The Every Body Book* (Simon, 2020) which includes what the author calls a 'special section' about gender dysphoria. For older adolescents (and adults), I highly recommend the School of Sexuality Education,[3] whose aim is to ensure everyone has access to a complete and comprehensive sex, sexuality and relationships education. Their approach is rights-based, sex-positive, non-binary and trauma-informed. Their recently published book *Sex Ed: An inclusive teenage guide to sex and relationships* (School of Sexuality Education, 2021) is refreshingly no holds barred.

Netflix and chill

From their descriptions of sex, Lane seemed emotionally cut-off from the physical experiences, almost as if they weren't a part of them. I had no sense of any enjoyment or sexual gratification. I knew that they detested their body 'from the neck down', and so I thought it must have been difficult, if not impossible, for them to associate their hated body with any pleasurable feelings. I took a risk and asked what, if anything, Lane found sexually satisfying. Their answer was direct.

'Wanking.'
'Wanking?'
'Yeah, wanking.'
'Is it okay to say more?'
'With Greb.'

The conversation was uncharacteristically stilted, and I could sense Lane's unease. I checked in with them, 'Is it okay to talk about this with me?'

'Yeah, it's fine. I just don't really know what to say.'
'You can say anything.'
'What do you want to know?'
'Well, I'm curious about your sexual relationships and what sex is like for you.'
'Okay.' They remained hesitant.
'You've mentioned wanking and you've mentioned Greb. How

---

3. https://schoolofsexed.org/

would you describe him?'

'Well, he's not my boyfriend, if that's what you mean. He's just a friend.'

'Just a friend who you wank with.' I smiled, in an attempt to lighten the heaviness, and to my relief, Lane smiled too.

'Yeah, a friend who I wank with.'

'What's he like?'

'He's bisexual. He mostly goes with boys.'

It was an interesting answer. I hadn't asked Lane how Greb identified sexually, and I don't think that's what I'd been wondering about either, but Lane had given me his sexual label. I assumed, therefore, that this must be an important element for Lane, and I attempted to explore it further.

'Greb's mostly attracted to boys.'

'Yeah.'

'And he's attracted to you.'

'I'm not sure…'

'You're not sure?'

'No.'

'How come?'

'I don't know. He's never said, and I've never really thought about it.'

'But you have sex together.'

'Yeah.'

'Isn't that a clue that he might be attracted to you?'

'Maybe.'

'Are you attracted to him?'

'I don't know.'

'You don't know?'

'No.'

'But you have sex together. You wank.'

'Yeah.'

I was sounding like a stuck record. The conversation was stuck. Lane seemed stuck, unable to answer (what seemed like) straightforward questions about whether they and Greb were sexually attracted to each other. I needed to change tack, put Greb to one side and explore the physical, sexual act itself.

'Can you tell me about the wanking?' It felt like a brave move on my part.

'What?' Lane seemed uncertain.

'The wanking. What's it like? I'm interested. And in what else you and Greb do?'

'Okay. This is weird. Well, we've kissed.'

'And...'

'Not much. It's not something we do very much.'

'The kissing?'

'Yeah.'

'Okay.'

'Usually, we just lie on the bed and watch Netflix.'

'Netflix and chill?'

Lane smiled at the reference, which we both recognised as a euphemism for sex. 'Yeah, Netflix and chill.'

'Okay.' I smiled too. The tension had been reduced by humour again, one of the most valuable tools in my arsenal when I'm working with adolescents, and Lane seemed more relaxed as they continued, 'I like holding his penis. I like the feel of it.'

'It feels nice?'

'It does, yeah.'

Lane told me they enjoyed the sensation of holding Greb's penis and they were fascinated by their ability to stroke it into an erect state. I wondered whether Greb ever masturbated Lane. They said he never did because they didn't like to be touched 'down there'. Lane said that sometimes Greb touched himself, or guided Lane's hand to his 'dick and balls' to show them what felt nice. So, the principal site of all sexual pleasure was the penis; more specifically Greb's penis. The way Lane described it, I didn't have a sense of Greb as a selfish sexual partner, or one who was taking advantage of Lane. My sense was of the sexual act as being comfortable, sensual and satisfying, but I had no sense of it as *sexually* gratifying. There wasn't much kissing or caressing, there was no penetration, no mutual masturbation and no sexual climax.

Although the sexual act was focused on someone else's penis, the sense I had was of a self-soothing act, as if the two bodies were merged, and as if Lane was perhaps simulating masturbation of their own (disavowed) penis. I'd previously had a sense of them as emotionally cut-off from the physical experience of sex, but now I had a sense of the male sex organ as being cut off (symbolically) from their body and presented as an appendage of Greb's. I was reminded of the concepts of animus (the masculine within the feminine) and anima (the feminine within the masculine), which, according to Jungian psychology, are abstract symbols or 'archetypes' of the unconscious mind (Jung, 1968). I had rarely experienced Lane presenting so peacefully in session. I could only imagine, therefore, that the masturbatory act itself must feel sublime.

Sublimation and semantics

I thought about the word 'sublime' and its similarity to the word 'sublimation'. I was playing with semantics, which I often do. Sometimes I do it out loud with the young person in session, as in our exploration of 'fine' or 'pan' or 'Netflix and chill', but frequently the playing with words happens in my mind, as part of my own reflection and processing. The way a person chooses this word over that one, and how they join them together to form language, is fascinating to me. The words that I choose are interesting too, both as a psychotherapist and as a writer. I was curious that the word 'sublime' had entered my awareness and the link I'd made with 'sublimation', which, in psychological terms, is a defence mechanism involving the expression of a strong desire or feeling, in a way that is deemed to be more socially acceptable.

Contemporary psychodynamic theory suggests that sublimation is a conscious process, adapted to enhance pleasure and feelings of control (Vaillant, 1994). As I've earlier explained, sublimation acts to integrate conflicting emotions and thoughts and transform unhelpful emotions or instincts into healthy ones. I wondered how these theories might help me to think about Lane and their seemingly sublime sexual experiences. Was the act of masturbation an act of sublimation? Had it become a way of transforming undesirable thoughts and feelings about their own body into more socially acceptable behaviours towards another? Possibly.

Me, myself and I

When Lane and I met again, we didn't talk about sex or sublimation, but we did talk about semantics. I'd been looking back through my process notes – the things I jot down after a session that strike me as interesting or unusual, or curious – ideas I might use as prompts, or thoughts I might want to think about some more, either in session or in supervision. I don't use people's names in my notes, as an extra precaution to protect their confidentiality; I just use an initial and the date of the session. Looking through my notes, I observed my use of M for Melanie in the referral and consultation and L for Lane from session two onwards. I reflected on the names, or rather the semantics of the names, and I realised, for the first time, what had been split off from the deadname[4] Melanie to make the preferred name Lane – the letters M, E and I: ME and I! When I shared this observation with Lane, they were as amazed as I was.

'I deleted myself. I got rid of me!'
'And I.'
'Yes, me and I.'
'I wonder where those parts of you went?'
'I think I killed them off.'
'You killed them off, along with your deadname?'
'Yeah, that's a good point.'
'Is that how you think of it?'
'Yeah, I think so. I think those parts of me died with Melanie.'
'And now?'
'I'm maybe ready to let parts of them back in.'

I think Lane was talking about their readiness for reintegration. The acknowledgment of the fragmented name provided a stark symbolism for Lane's fragmented sense of self. They came to therapy feeling unstable, not knowing who they were or how they identified, which caused them to feel anxious, withdrawn and overwhelmed. They gave accounts of a topsy-turvy, upside-down existence, where nothing made sense, and everything was merged, blurred or borrowed. My first observation about Lane was to do with a lack of self-care and that the way they presented didn't make sense. With hindsight, I think they were presenting a false self because they didn't know what was authentically them. Winnicott introduced the concepts of false self (a defence) and true self, which is based on lived experience and feeling real (Winnicott, 1965a).

On reflection, Lane's sense of self seemed unstable because their personality was fragmented – a component of ordinary adolescence, compounded by their experience (Kohut, 1971). Themes of boundary testing, fragmentation and projection were played out in therapy,

---

4. The term deadname refers to a person's birth name that they no longer use. If you know their name, you should use it, and if you're unsure, you should ask. Using a deadname (deadnaming) when you know a person's name is disrespectful and akin to misgendering (Holleb, 2019).

inevitably, due to the tendency to unconsciously act out experiences from the past in the present (Freud, 1920). These defensive repetition compulsions were demonstrated by both Lane and Gill. With one foot in the therapeutic relationship and one foot outside it, I could notice, process and work through, rather than get blindly drawn into playing out the familiar themes of erratic relationships, disloyalty, ambivalence, ambiguity and a lack of boundaries.

I was able to offer a safe, consistent, reliable space that Lane could come to and leave each week, or not, as they chose. I monitored Lane's self-injury without over- or under-reacting, and tried to make sense of it with them. I acknowledged their sexual experiences, without over- or under-reacting, and tried to make sense of them too. Some of my sense-making was internal, informed by psychoanalytic theory; some of it was done collaboratively with Lane. Together, we arrived at a place where we recognised the fragmented parts of the self – conscious and unconscious, anima and animus, symbolic and lived reality, gender and sexuality, me and I – so that the process of reintegration could begin and so that Lane could be their true, authentic self.

5

Wanking

Reggie is a child in care with an unusual sexual fetish that keeps leading to rejection. Can psychotherapy help him to understand the links between his early developmental experiences and his adolescent sexual compulsion, so that he can break the cycle of repetition?

. . . .

Reggie was referred to me for psychotherapy by his social worker. The lengthy referral contained factual and demographic information, such as date of birth, current and previous addresses, and current and previous schools. I remember reading it and feeling that I had no sense of who Reggie was. This was not surprising, given that the social worker who made the referral was new in post and had never actually met him. Reggie, on the other hand, had been in the care system since the age of six. But, on reviewing her newly acquired case files, the social worker noticed that he had not received any therapeutic support.

The number of children in long-term care who have not had any kind of therapeutic input is alarming. There are many reasons for this: sometimes the young person refuses help, and sometimes it is not offered. Often, young people in care are moved around so frequently that they are never in one place long enough to engage in therapy. It makes sense to wait until a young person is settled in their placement before therapy is offered, because they need a secure enough base to feel contained enough to access therapy. If they're not settled at home, they will find it hard to settle in therapy. But many children in care are moved so frequently from placement to placement that they are never anywhere long enough to feel settled and, consequently, they never receive any therapeutic support.

Another issue is funding. Therapy is perceived as expensive, and for children who are looked after outside of the placing authority's local area, the fees can be even more costly. The amounts charged by NHS trusts for each appointment that a young 'out-of-area' person has with their child and adolescent mental health services (CAMHS) makes private therapy a much more cost-effective solution. Which is why the referring social worker decided that this was the best option for Reggie and sent him to me.

By way of introduction, she shared a document with me that detailed Reggie's family history. I learned that he had witnessed domestic violence in his early years and that his alcohol-dependent father had eventually left the family home when Reggie was four. His mother misused substances and had bouts of severe depression. She had been offered support to help her to parent Reggie and his two younger siblings but had found it difficult to engage with professionals. After numerous failed attempts to support the family, all three children were eventually placed on a Full Care Order (FCO) and sent to separate foster placements in different parts of the country.

The referring social worker requested an 'urgent' assessment of Reggie, who was presenting as 'difficult to manage' in his current placement, which, she said, was at risk of breaking down. Both the social worker and the foster carer thought that Reggie would benefit from 'anger management', which made me cringe. I frequently receive requests for this type of 'treatment', usually for boys, often boys in care, and it irritates me. It implies an underlying assumption that the young person needs their anger fixed, when they usually have plenty to be angry about. I offered to meet Reggie, to assess his therapeutic needs and to find out if he wanted to engage in psychotherapy; whatever I or the social worker thought about his needs, it should be his choice.

First impressions

I met Reggie in the week after his 16th birthday, which, he told me, had come and gone without much celebration. For initial sessions, I invite the young person to attend with their parent or carer, but Reggie specifically requested to come alone, and I agreed to meet him unaccompanied. Just like the 'if', the 'who' and 'how' and 'when' of therapy should be the young person's choice, and I remember feeling pleased that he was able to assert himself, but curious about why he chose to come alone. It's important for me to make a relationship with carers too, so that they are linked into what happens in therapy, and I wondered why Reggie wanted to keep us separate. But for now, I thought it was important to respect his wishes, with a view to inviting the carer to a later appointment. I also wondered if Reggie was communicating that he could look after himself, and this particularly interested me, given that he was a 'looked-after' child.

When I opened the door to Reggie, the first thing that struck me was that he was black; I hadn't been informed about his ethnicity. In my experience, this apparent 'colour blindness' is not unusual when white social workers place black children in placements with white families or refer black children to white therapists, such as me. I find this concerning. To ignore the colour of someone's skin, or claim not to see it, seems dismissive; it's like saying, 'I haven't seen *you*'. I live and work in a part of the UK with limited but thankfully growing diversity, which means I come across this situation a lot in my work with children in care, who have been placed here from parts of the country where there are bigger populations of ethnic minority groups. I think it's important to be 'colour conscious' (aware of colour) and to open up an exploration of these themes in the therapy room.

Reggie was dressed comfortably in jeans, jumper and high-end trainers, his hair neatly styled. I noted that he seemed to take pride in his appearance. Everything about Reggie's presentation made him appear older than his 16 years. He was tall and well built. He sank into the sofa and sat with his legs wide apart, one arm slung over the back, the other hanging loosely in front of his groin. He looked me directly in the eye, smiled widely and said, 'Hi, I'm Reggie.' It was as charming a welcome as I could imagine.

Reggie's body language was very open, and I wondered what this might portray about how he would engage in therapy specifically, and how he related to other people in the real world more generally. I also wondered if he would have presented differently if his foster carer had been there with us. As we made our introductions and discussed the therapeutic contract, I noticed that Reggie pushed his sleeves up to the elbow, showing off his toned forearms. He also repeatedly adjusted his crotch, holding his groin with his right hand and wriggling about in a way I could not help but notice. I wondered whether his fidgeting was a sign of nerves or something sexual. At some level, Reggie wanted me to notice that he was a sexually mature young man with a muscular physique and a penis.

I find it useful to notice my initial thoughts and feelings in response to a new client the first time we meet. This helps to inform my working hypothesis and any initial clinical formulations. The first point of significance was that the glaringly obvious fact of Reggie's ethnicity had not been communicated to me in the referral. This made me wonder what else might have been withheld by the system. I also noted that Reggie seemed to bring something sexual into the room that it was impossible for me to ignore.

The normal stuff

I invited Reggie to tell me about himself and why he was here. He cautioned, 'I might *seem* like a normal teenager. Well, I am a teenager and there are some things about me that are normal...'

I nodded my understanding and encouraged him to go on.

'I'm good at sport, especially football. I'm doing well in my lessons. I'm popular at school and I have lots of friends. People like me – especially the girls,' he added, with that charming smile he'd greeted me with earlier.

'It makes you smile to know the girls like you,' I commented.

'Yeah, it feels good, you know?'

I wasn't sure I did know. I wasn't sure what Reggie was actually communicating to me. Was he flirting with me or warning me off? There was a confusing kind of push/pull feeling to the way he was relating to me. I could well believe his popularity: a good-looking, confident and sporty young man would no doubt attract a lot of female attention. I wondered what he did with that attention once he had it, and I wondered too what he would do with my full-on, focused, individual attention here. Would he be able to handle it? Might Reggie struggle with an intimate therapeutic relationship? Picking up on what he'd said about seeming normal, I asked if he could say more about that.

'The normal stuff is the sport, the girls, my friends, you know?'

'Yes, I know, the stuff you've already told me about. But it seems there's something else?'

'Yes, the abnormal bit.'

'Abnormal?'

'The wanking.'

'The wanking? That sounds normal enough, Reggie.'

'Not the way I do it. For me, it's a fetish.'

'A fetish?'

'Yeah. I have to dress up while I wank; it really turns me on.'

I was struck by his vocabulary. Did 16-year-olds really use words like 'fetish' and 'turned on'? I certainly hadn't heard them do so with such confidence during a first meeting with an adult. Again, I simply nodded my encouragement for Reggie to continue. In the first 20 minutes of our first session, he told me that he dressed up in women's clothes as an aid to masturbation and that he did this about five out of seven days every week. I wondered about the significance of this disclosure and asked Reggie if it was something that bothered him, and if it was something that he wanted to change.

'It doesn't really bother me, but it bothers other people.'

'Who does it bother?' I enquired.

'The carers.'

'I'm wondering what your wanking has got to do with your carers.'

'Quite a lot, apparently. It's the reason I've had so many placements.'

'How many?'

'Thirteen. This is number 14.'

'I'm sorry to hear that, Reggie. That's a lot of moving around and disruption.'

'It's not your fault.'

'Is it anyone's fault?'

'Mine, apparently.'

'Because of the wanking?'

'Yes, because of the wanking.'

Reggie told me that the reason that each one of his previous placements had broken down was because the foster carers had discovered his 'habit'. I was interested in his language and wondered to myself who had perceived Reggie's fetishistic masturbation as habitual. Aloud, I asked why his foster carers didn't know about it before he moved somewhere new. He told me that 'they' (social services) never shared it with any of the families prior to them accepting him in placement. Here was something else that hadn't been shared with me: first, Reggie's ethnicity, which was the first thing I'd observed, and now his fetish, which had been one of the first things that he'd shared. Actually, it was more than shared, it was more like unburdened.

The withholding of information bothered me more than Reggie's disclosure, and I felt a surge of anger on his behalf that he had been repeatedly set up to fail in numerous placements. My feeling response reminded me that the therapy referral had requested 'anger management'. I shared this with Reggie, and he said it pissed him off that people thought of him as 'another angry black man who needed anger management'. We smiled at the irony and it felt like we had made a connection.

I asked him, '*Are* you an angry black man, Reggie?'

'Not in the way they make out.'

'It makes me think about what you said earlier about being a "normal teenager" and that you *are* a teenager and there *are* some things about you that are normal…'

'And I *am* a black man and sometimes I get angry, don't get me wrong, but I'm *not* an "angry black man".'

'And it's frustrating that you would be perceived that way.'

'Yeah.'

The abnormality

Clients communicate by impact as well as words, and my initial response to Reggie was profound. I felt an immediate and heavy weight of responsibility: to make our contract explicit, to neither condemn nor condone his sexual behaviour and to use his words rather than my own to describe it. Of course, these obligations characterise every client encounter, but with Reggie they felt much more critical. It is likely that I was responding to a complicated mix of Reggie's physical presentation as well as his own internal feelings. Looking back, I don't think I wanted to admit to myself, as much as to Reggie, that I was shocked by his overt and unusual sexual presentation, but I suppose I must have been, and it's difficult for me to admit that even now.

Reggie told me he had googled various themes to do with his behaviour, typing *fetish*, *wanking* and *dressing up in women's clothes* into search engines. He said that what he discovered online disgusted him and that the images he saw had assured him that he wasn't gay or a transvestite and that, 'no offence, I don't want to be a woman either'. Reggie was telling me about how he had turned to the internet in an attempt to understand his behaviour. I wondered if he was now turning to me to help him to understand, and who I would turn to for guidance and support. His research had proved counterproductive because it left him feeling 'abnormal' and 'perverted' because he was unable to find anyone online who liked what he liked.

I was struck by what seemed like Reggie's maturity in wanting to make sense of himself and I had a strong urge to reassure him that he was not abnormal or perverted. I felt a dilemma in how best to respond and was acutely aware of not wanting to say the wrong thing – and that I had no idea what the 'right' thing might be. I picked up on his use of the terms 'abnormal' and 'perverse' and said that 'unusual' might be better. I very much needed to change the punishing adjectives Reggie used to describe himself to ones that felt less judgemental. Again, with hindsight, I think I was searching for words that would feel more comfortable to me. His behaviour could legitimately be described as abnormal and perverse. My attempts to normalise it demonstrated, I think, how hard it was for me to stay with the feelings of uncomfortable-ness and confusion, just as it must have been hard for Reggie. The sexual fetish was hard to think about, and that was exactly what Reggie had invited me to do.

He accepted my offer of six individual sessions to see if I could help him to make sense of his behaviour. I let his foster carer and social worker know, and they agreed with the plan. None of us mentioned anger management.

In search of meaning

In the next session, I encouraged Reggie to tell me about the feelings evoked by dressing up. He described feeling turned on and sexy. He fidgeted on the couch and adjusted his crotch in a way that was obvious, and which again appeared to be tinged with sexual excitement. When I asked, he confirmed that thinking about the fetish turned him on too, but not to the same extent as acting it out. He told me, 'I haven't got a hard on right now!' and I was relieved to hear it. I'm not sure how I'd have reacted if he'd said that he had. He also admitted that recently he had given in to the impulse to cover his entire body, including his face, with female clothing before masturbating to a climax inside it.

Reggie spoke openly and confidently, with the air of an adult. It often felt as if he was flirting with me or attempting to seduce me, and that he enjoyed the sense of potency this gave him. I'm not suggesting that this was conscious or intentional, or that Reggie *actually* wanted to seduce me, but I think I was picking up a communication that perhaps belonged to another relationship. In therapy jargon, this was erotic transference, meaning that characteristics of a relationship with someone else had been transferred onto me. So, it *felt* as if Reggie was trying to seduce me, but in fact he was communicating (unconsciously) something about his wish to seduce someone else. The only inkling of discomfort apparent from Reggie as he spoke was related to his choice of *female* clothing as a source of sexual gratification, and this is what made it seem significant. I wondered what his choice might represent, at a symbolic level, and encouraged Reggie to join me on an exploration of its hidden meaning. I asked him to tell me about the types of clothing he used, including where and how he sourced them. He needed to be specific and detailed if we were going to make sense of it.

Reggie said he 'borrowed' clothing from his carer. She had some nightdresses that he especially liked, because they felt silky and were big enough for him to get inside, but once he'd finished with them, they were difficult to dispose of. I wondered how on earth a young man might secretly dispose of a borrowed nightie covered in semen. He said he usually shoved it in the washing machine and hoped it would go unnoticed among the regular laundry. On a day-to-day basis though, he said he mostly used smaller garments like knickers or silky socks or tights, which he could more easily hide. He usually took them from his carer but admitted also to occasional shoplifting.

Reggie described how it was possible to get parts of himself inside the smaller garments or parts of himself inside different garments at the same time. I checked back with him my sense that the sensation of the fabric was important, as was the ability to wrap himself, or parts of himself, inside it. He said yes. I checked that what I had heard him say was that he took items of female underwear and put them on his penis as well as on other parts of his body, including his face. He agreed. And I checked that he did this almost every day because it turned him on and enabled him to masturbate to a climax. Reggie said yes, I had understood correctly everything he'd told me.

There was no doubt that what he vividly described was a sexual fetish. According to the dictionary definition, a fetish is 'a sexual interest in an object', or, 'an activity or object that you are so interested in that you spend an unreasonable amount of time thinking about it or doing it' (Cambridge Dictionary, 2021).

Origins of fetishism

It is difficult for me to think about sex and fetishes without referencing Freud, who defined fetishism as the 'unsuitable substitute for the sexual object' (Freud, 1905). The prevailing question in my mind was whether Reggie's fetish was 'unsuitable'. We needed to explore further. When I met him again, I wondered if he could remember the first time he had used a female garment as a fetish object. He remembered very clearly an event that happened when he was six years old and in his first foster placement. Sissy, the biological daughter of his foster carers, was about 16 – the same age as Reggie was now. He recalled her treating him with a mixture of contempt and titillation, parading around the house, 'flaunting herself', which six-year-old Reggie must have found quite tantalising, having never come across a teenage girl before. When Sissy went out, which she often did, he would creep into the forbidden territory of her bedroom and sneak a peek at her things. At first his interest was limited to the items on display – posters of actors and boybands, glossy magazines, make-up and trinkets – things that were typically girly and unknown to him. But Reggie's curiosity about the aloof adolescent he shared a home with soon led him into her cupboards and drawers to explore what lay there.

Reggie said he liked the feel of Sissy's clothes and the way they smelled, which was very different to his own garments and aroma, of course. He described taking things from her drawers and rubbing them on his skin: first his face and then his chest. He admitted it became a 'bit of a thing' and soon he couldn't wait for her to go out so that he could get his hands on her stuff. Sometimes he took things and put them under his pillow so he could hold them next to himself in bed at night. Reggie told me that Sissy must have rumbled him, because drawings of frilly knickers began to appear on his books, which 'embarrassed the hell' out of him. He knew that she had done it, and *she* knew that *he* knew, and that he wouldn't say anything because his 'crime' was much worse than hers. By that point, Reggie's curiosity had developed from fingering Sissy's underwear to putting it on so that he could experience what it felt like to be inside it. He said, very quietly, that it had felt nice.

It brought to my mind the transition many heterosexual adolescent boys make from platonic attraction based on how a girl looks on the outside to an exploration of the insides of girls' bodies, initially through digital and eventually penis-in-vagina penetration.

The atmosphere in the therapy room felt different. Reggie himself seemed different. I had more of a sense of an emotionally immature little boy than a sexually developed young man. Gone was the sexual charge that had accompanied Reggie's previous descriptions of his sexual behaviour. This was something more sensitive and cosseting. We thought together about the distinction between comfort and sexual pleasure, and I suggested that the two feelings were perhaps not so dissimilar in their origins. To his credit, Reggie was willing to contemplate my suggestion – that, while the label he attached to his feelings had changed – from nice/comforting to turned on/fetish – the physical feeling he got now might not be so dissimilar to that experienced by his six-year-old younger self.

Infantile sexuality is a complex notion, the significance of which Freud first explored in *The Aetiology of Hysteria* (Freud, 1896), an interesting title given the hysterical reactions Reggie's behaviour appeared to provoke among professionals. Freud proposed that infantile libido developed in one of three directions: normal sexual life, neurosis or perversion. Sexual impulses that originate during childhood are often repressed, while those that are acted out can appear as sexual perversions throughout adolescence and into adulthood.

Reggie had repeatedly used the word 'perverse' to describe his behaviour, which I found uncomfortable. With more context to his story, I was beginning to understand where this view of himself might have originated. Reggie's earliest experience of dressing up presented a double-edged sword. On the one hand, it was sensual and comforting; on the other, it was ridiculed by his female witness. Might it be that Reggie's continued auto-erotic behaviour represented a search for the pleasurable sensations that he had initially experienced and remembered and which he now longed to replicate? I was also curious about the feelings of humiliation and the possibility that they were part of the turn-on for Reggie now. I knew I would need to tread carefully to explore this possibility further.

Seeking pleasure/disavowing pain

As therapy progressed, Reggie's bravado diminished. He admitted to a fear that his behaviour would land him in a 'mad house'. He expressed his dilemma by telling me that he needed my help to make the guilty voice in his head louder and the sexual voice quieter. I recognised this as his desire to fulfil the external demands being placed upon him at the expense of his own internal sexual impulses. I also recognised a classic psychological dilemma between the instincts of the pleasure-seeking id and those of the conscientious superego. I wondered about the guilty (superego) voice and Reggie admitted to feeling enormous shame after he reached climax. Hearing Reggie's honest accounts of his sexual urges, I had the sense that his behaviour had an addictive quality. Indeed, the first time we had thought together about his fetish, he had referred to it as a 'habit'.

I also recalled the details of Reggie's family history. His parents were both addicts: his mother abused substances and his father was dependent on alcohol. It's not a straightforward case of cause and effect, but a family history of addiction is a risk factor for addiction and for behavioural difficulties, which in turn can increase the risk of addictive behaviours (National Institute on Drug Abuse, 2011). So, perhaps Reggie had inherited a genetic predisposition towards addiction. I thought that might go some way towards explaining his behaviour, but it would not help us to understand the *nature* of his fetish. I was mindful of the proposition, from my reading of psychoanalytic literature, that, 'objects of desire perform the function of a drug' (McDougall, 1995, p.183), and that the purpose of any addictive behaviour is to dispel painful feelings. Put very simply, I thought that Reggie might masturbate in order to make himself feel better.

But the pervasiveness of his fetish, despite his fear of institutionalisation and the reality of abandonment by his foster carers, suggested an additional psychological function that required ongoing exploration. When people do things that are potentially destructive, there has to be a reason. Often that reason is unconscious, and the search for it can be the stuff of long-term psychotherapy.

Reggie was able to identify numerous triggers for dressing up and masturbating in women's clothing. These included boredom and anxiety, as well as feeling turned on; all very ordinary feelings for a 16-year-old young man to be feeling. He told me that the greatest levels of anxiety created the greatest compulsion to cover his whole body with female garments. So, the behaviour seemed to be a way of getting rid of the anxious feelings. I think that was happening in therapy too. Sometimes, I turn to psychodynamic literature to help me understand what might be going on for a young person – and sometimes it is a way to contain my own anxiety. I was aware, while working with Reggie, that I was relying on theory much more than I ordinarily would; I was intellectualising rather than feeling. I remembered what he had told me about his own attempts to understand his behaviour by searching the internet. The temptation to intellectualise, to think rather than feel, can be a psychological defence. I was struck by the parallels in our behaviour: it was as if something of Reggie's struggle to make theoretical sense of his behaviour and disavow the feelings had been projected onto me. I realised that I needed to make space for feeling as well as thinking, for both of us; however uncomfortable that might be for both of us too.

Psychoanalytic theory suggests that the addictive object fulfils a soothing function that the individual is unable to provide for him or herself. This lent support to my hypothesis that Reggie's choice of female garments was significant and perhaps provided a symbolic connection to the person who they represented and replaced. Due to Reggie's family background, it is likely that he had learnt to rely on self-soothing strategies from early infancy, because his parents would not have been available to fulfil this function and provide comfort for their baby, due to their own addictions. It seems plausible to deduce, therefore, that Reggie's impulse to be covered by and get inside female garments represented an unconscious desire to get inside and be held by the mother who had abandoned him. In other words, the behaviour was communicating a feeling.

Paradoxically, it was this very desire to be mothered that caused Reggie to be repeatedly abandoned by subsequent mother substitutes. In my work I see a lot of what can be recognised as 'repetition compulsion' (Freud, 1920). Put simply, Reggie was likely to continue repeating the same behaviour until he was able to understand it. And the only way to understand it would be to acknowledge the feelings and bring the unconscious motivation into conscious awareness.

Reggie had told me that there was nothing that made him feel as good as masturbating inside an item of female clothing. However, he also acknowledged that nothing made him feel as guilty as he did after climaxing in this way. Perhaps the reason that his compulsion had ultimately failed him so far was because it represented a somatic rather than a psychological attempt to deal with his anxiety. In other words, in order to change his behaviour, if that was what he wanted to do, he needed to make sense of it psychologically.

Mothers

Reggie craved a stable home and a mother (or mother substitute) to take care of him, but his placements had been repeatedly jeopardised by the discovery of, and lack of understanding about, his habitual fetish. Since the loss of his own mother, he had lost 13 replacement mothers and was now residing with his 14th. He told me that he did not have the willpower to change, but that a part of him hoped that I could help him. I tried to explain that, while I could carry on thinking with him, I could not change him and would not try. I said that I hoped I would be able to help him to feel more in control of his masturbation fantasies so that his behaviour could be less compulsive. This was difficult for me to communicate to Reggie because he viewed psychotherapy as a last chance 'cure' that would prevent abandonment by his current foster carer, whom he said he liked very much. Reggie felt that she had demonstrated that she wanted the placement to work by supporting his referral to me for help rather than just kicking him out when she discovered his behaviour.

Reggie repeatedly told me how supportive she was, and I had a sense that he idealised her. I wondered if it was wishful thinking on his part; that he wanted to believe that he had finally found the ideal mother who had eluded him all of his life. I also wondered what substance there was to this and asked Reggie if he could say more about the support she provided that previous foster carers had denied him. He told me that she checked his room every day for women's clothing and reminded him that, if she found any, he would have to leave. Was this tough love? To me, it sounded persecutory rather than supportive. I feared for the longevity of the placement and was curious to know more about Reggie's relationship with his foster carer.

I thought that the way Reggie related to me might provide some insight into how he related to other 'mothers' – transference, again, or more specifically, maternal transference. Reggie often told me that he had opened up to me more than he had to anyone else before. He said that he trusted me and that our sessions were really helping him. I hoped that he did trust me and that the sessions were helping, but I have learned to look beyond the face value of verbal communications such as these, which can be attempts at flattery. I could well imagine Reggie intimating to his carer that she was the ideal foster carer and better than any other foster carer who had come before her. Maybe he thought that if she thought that he really believed that, she would be unable to reject him because such a good 'mother' would never do such a treacherous thing. But, of course, Reggie's attempts were doomed to failure because he would never find a good enough substitute for the mother he lost in infancy and whom he longed to replace.

I have experienced how attempts to make one person feel more special or more knowing than another can have the effect of inhibiting open communication between professionals and carers. I had seen for myself the inhibited communication between professionals throughout Reggie's experience, and have noticed in general how this tends to happen most often when clients have unusual and complex needs – the very cases where effective communication is most important. I wondered if Reggie's flattery and tendency to idealise could therefore represent another repetition compulsion and a further jeopardy to the stability of his placement by 'splitting' the professionals.

Splitting describes the way a person views things, people or experiences in binary terms, such as good/bad, and is another (unconscious) attempt at psychological defence. In the transference, Reggie was telling me what I needed to do: it was time for me to meet his foster carer. I checked this out with Reggie and thought with him about what we would and would not share with her. Therapy sessions are confidential, and I would take my lead from him. I invited June, his foster carer, to join us the following week so that we could think together about how the sessions were going and where they might go from here.

Whose problem is it, anyway?

June was in her late middle age. She was not particularly smiley, and I did not especially warm to her. I thought she seemed a bit detached. I am aware that my description of her certainly illustrates the detachment I felt that first time I met her. When I thanked her for accompanying Reggie to the session, she said she didn't really understand why I had asked her to come. I felt as if she were saying, 'This is his problem, not mine.' In a way she was right, of course, but if Reggie was going to remain in her care, potentially into early adulthood, I believed she should share some of the responsibility that was currently weighing heavily on his shoulders.

I explained to June that we had spent the sessions so far thinking about Reggie's sexual behaviour. She visibly winced and it was evident that sex was difficult for her to think and talk about. It amazes me how many professionals working with adolescents can't think or talk about sex when it's pretty much all adolescents think and talk about pretty much most of the time. I proceeded gently and reiterated what I had explained to Reggie several times before: that my role was to help him to understand his behaviour so that he could feel more in control of it.

June asked me directly if I could make him stop wanking. She didn't use the word 'wanking', she just sort of intimated towards his crotch with her head. I said that I would not attempt to do that but that if Reggie wanted to change his behaviour, then learning what it might be about would be a good place to start. June relaxed a bit, and we were able to continue.

She said she was angry that she hadn't known about Reggie's 'habit' before he came to live with her. I acknowledged that this was a perfectly understandable response, but also pointed out that this was not Reggie's fault. It felt important that Reggie heard me say that and for June to acknowledge that it was true. I was keen to direct any projected anger away from Reggie to where it more reasonably belonged, which was with the professional system. I asked June when she discovered Reggie's habit, and she said she had found some of her clothes stuffed in the bathroom bin, wrapped in tissues. Again, I reassured June that her feelings of shock and repulsion were perfectly understandable.

As agreed with Reggie, I explained to June that he didn't feel in control of how and how often he masturbated, but that he had expressed a desire to change that. I shared that he had demonstrated a commitment to therapy and was using the sessions well. I explained that, together, we were beginning to understand where his sexual behaviour might have originated but this was going to take a while longer to fully comprehend. June seemed satisfied. I also felt that it was important to highlight our different roles and responsibilities in supporting Reggie. Mine was to provide a thinking space and also, it seemed, to help facilitate Reggie's relationship with June. June's role was to care for him and meet his basic needs and she seemed to be doing a good enough job of this. I use the term 'good enough' deliberately, but not to denigrate: no mother can be perfect, and good enough is good enough. By the way, the same goes for psychotherapists, as I've said before, but it's good to be reminded.

The next part of the review was to encourage June and Reggie to form a mutually acceptable contract. Sometimes in my work I find it necessary to be more directive than usual, and this was one of those occasions. I suggested that June should respect Reggie's private space in her home. I suggested that she provide him with a bin for his room, which he would be responsible for emptying and keeping clean. He could dispose of whatever he needed to in the bin, without fear of reprisal. In return, Reggie would have to agree that he would not enter June's bedroom or take any of her things. This basic agreement reinstated the boundaries around roles, responsibilities, respect for private spaces and behaviour, in the interests of both Reggie and June. They both relaxed as we discussed this and agreed to abide by the new contract. We set a date for a further review meeting in six weeks' time as it felt important to keep June included in the therapeutic process and on board in supporting Reggie.

Ending

In the individual session following the review, Reggie announced that he had only masturbated in female clothes twice that week and that this was a record. He added mischievously that he had masturbated 'in the normal way' a couple of times too. When I remarked that Reggie seemed pleased, his demeanour immediately altered. He told me he *was* pleased and wondered why I wasn't pleased too. This, to me, was an expression of his need to please me, as well as his sense of rejection that he had seemingly failed to do so. I understood this as a transference communication about Reggie's need to please a whole line of disapproving mothers before me. In his experience, things were either good or bad, and his behaviour was perceived as either pleasing or displeasing. He expected one of two responses and the absence of approval could only mean disapproval, in Reggie's mind. The former meant he could stay and be cared for while the latter preceded abandonment.

My relationship with Reggie had become comfortable over the initial period of psychotherapy and we had established an easy rapport. While this reassured me that we had a safe and secure enough relationship, it was apparent now that Reggie's defences were still too fragile for him to manage his constant fear of rejection. He was angry with me and he let me know it. He said he did not need to come to therapy any more and that I had done enough to help him. He said he was on his own now and that it was down to him to sort himself out. He left the session early and said he would not be coming back. I was shocked and hurt and felt responsible for hurting Reggie.

I considered his parting words as they continued to echo around the empty space left by his early departure. '*You've done enough. I'm on my own. It's down to me.*' I reflected on what I had done and whether it had been enough. I thought we had made considerable headway into understanding the origins of Reggie's fetish and what it represented for him in the present. I also thought I had helped to facilitate a better relationship for Reggie with his foster carer, so that he could feel more understood by her and she could be in a stronger position to support him. Whether this was enough, only Reggie could say. He had spat out the words 'You've done enough', and I was taking them to mean the opposite – that I should have done more. However, on reflection, I thought there was a possibility that he had meant exactly what he had said, that I *had* done enough for him, for now. He had followed this with the statements, 'I'm on my own' and, 'It's down to me'. Again, it occurred to me that he might be right, that he might well be ready to do it on his own, and that he might be ready to end therapy. But I hoped it wouldn't be like this, angry and abrupt, which seemed to mirror the way his foster placements had ended, without thought or preparation.

During the following week I received a telephone call from June. She had never contacted me before and this was a highly significant communication. She told me that Reggie had come home from therapy upset that he had shouted at me and that he felt embarrassed about walking out. This had precipitated a long and honest conversation between Reggie and June about his sexual behaviour and he had broken down and cried with her for the first time since being in her care. When I asked what happened next, she told me that she held Reggie while he cried. She was telling me that she had mothered him and that he had allowed her to hold him, physically as well as symbolically. I felt very moved by the image of Reggie and June in a maternal embrace. June said she had told Reggie I would be okay about him walking out and encouraged him to return for his session with me the following week. He said that he would, but also told her that he didn't need any more therapy. I said he was probably right, he had June, and I asked her to convey to Reggie that I would look forward to seeing him at our regular time the following week and that we could think together about planning our ending.

Reggie attended five more sessions and we continued to think together about the main themes to do with his sexuality and relationships. But we also talked about some more ordinary aspects of adolescent life – the 'normal' stuff. Reggie started going out with a girl at school and was enjoying having female company. He admitted that he had been terrified of girls and had perceived them as threatening and intimidating and had tried to keep his distance from them. Unfortunately for Reggie, his aloofness had only added to his allure and made him appear even more attractive to the girls in his year group and beyond. Alice was different. She sounded nice. She was the same age as Reggie, and they were spending their time getting to know each other by hanging out in juice bars and going to the cinema together. He told me that they were both virgins and in no hurry to consummate their fledgling relationship. Reggie was enjoying the physical intimacy of cuddles and kisses and, according to him, Alice was too.

His relationship with June was on an even keel and she had demonstrated her commitment to Reggie by applying for 'permanency' – a legal process that cements a foster placement as permanent until a young person's 18th birthday. Possibly for the first time ever, Reggie had a sense of a secure and stable base and a good enough 'mother'. During our final therapy session, he told me that he could not remember the last time he masturbated in female clothing. He added, with a mischievous smile, that he still 'wanked the regular way' several times a week, and I told him that I was very pleased to hear it.

I reflected on the young black man with a fetish who had been sent to me for anger management, almost as a box-ticking exercise, to prevent another placement from breaking down. What had struck me the first time we met was what had been withheld from me by the professional system – the part about him being black, and the part about the fetish – which reduced him to another generic angry young man in care. This withholding from me had paralleled the withholding of information from each new foster carer and the sense of shame and secrecy that shrouded Reggie's sexual exploration.

The difficult-to-talk-and-think-about stuff, which had been split off in the system, had proved difficult to feel about too. Both Reggie and I had used intellectualisation as a defence. We'd got caught up in a process of repetition, and both erotic transference and, later, maternal transference had been played out in therapy. But I'd managed to notice the compulsion to repeat early on, so that it could be worked through. In just a dozen or so sessions of psychotherapy, thanks to Reggie's willingness to think and feel and my capacity to think and feel with him, and June's capacity to think and feel about him, we had traced the origins of his sexual behaviour back to infancy and to his desire to feel soothed and comforted by a 'mother'. We'd understood that it was this desire to be mothered that caused Reggie to repeat the sexual behaviour that, paradoxically, had resulted in him being repeatedly abandoned by 13 mother substitutes. And, once we'd understood, we were able to bring the unconscious motivation into conscious awareness, so that the behaviour was no longer addictive or habitual and his 14th (re-)placement 'mother' could be experienced as secure enough and good enough.

In my closing report to the social worker, I wrote that I had enjoyed helping Reggie to explore his sexual needs and desires in the context of his developmental history. I shared that he had engaged fully in the therapeutic process and had developed a greater understanding of his wishes and feelings. I was also able to share that Reggie felt comfortable and contained in his placement and that I supported the plan for him to remain in June's care. Finally, Reggie had been given the opportunity to recognise and accept a good enough mother and achieve reparation for his early experiences. I made no reference to anger management. Or wanking. That was Reggie's business.

6

Maturation

Maeve has low self-esteem. She might be depressed; she might have an eating disorder; she might have body dysmorphia; she might be at risk of suicide. How can therapy help Maeve to re-establish her sense of self, so that she can flourish into a young woman?

. . . .

As I've stated already, 16-year-old girls with low self-esteem make up a large proportion of my caseload. This presenting issue varies from a mild-to-moderate sense of not feeling good enough to a debilitating sense of worthlessness. For Maeve, the feeling was unbearable. She was a Year-11 student who had been achieving well academically until suddenly her grades started to decline, 'for no apparent reason'. At least, this is what I was told when I met Maeve and her mother, Fi, for the first time.

I don't buy the 'for no reason' line; there is always a reason, even if it's not immediately apparent. One of my tasks, as a psychotherapist, is to find out what the reason is, so that we can understand why the behaviour manifested in the first place, the purpose it serves (because there is always a purpose) and, hopefully, bring about change. That said, I don't see the goal of therapy as changing behaviour *per se*, but once it makes sense, change does happen, and change of some type or other is usually clients' desired outcome when they seek my help. Change is also the task of maturation – one of the primary tasks of adolescence. As the French philosopher Henri Bergson wrote: 'To exist is to change, to change is to mature, to mature is to go on creating oneself endlessly' (Bergson, 1983, p.7).

I see another of my tasks (sometimes) as encouraging more open, honest communication between a young person and their parent. This is one of the reasons I invite both parent(s) and child to the initial consultation and include the parent(s) in regular review meetings throughout the period of ongoing psychotherapy. Often, young people don't tell their parents what they're really doing or how they're really feeling, for a number of reasons, such as fear of reprisal or a desire not to upset them. In my experience, this withholding works both ways, with parents withholding how *they* really feel and what *they* really fear from their children too. These three-way (sometimes more) difficult conversations can feel awkward and intense for families, but by offering my support and a less emotional perspective, I aim to help parent(s) and child understand each other better, as my conversations with Fi and Maeve will, I hope, demonstrate.

The reason Fi had sought my help for her daughter was because Maeve had stopped attending school and going out socialising with friends. According to her mother, Maeve wasn't eating, was always sad and often argumentative, and spent most of her time in her room. Fi thought that Maeve was depressed and was worried that she might also be developing an eating disorder. When I asked what they wanted to be different, Fi said she wanted Maeve to be back at school, getting good grades in her GCSEs, socialising and eating 'normally' again. When I asked Maeve what she wanted, she said, 'Not to feel like this.' It is not unusual for young people with low self-esteem to display features of low mood, and Maeve certainly presented in this way. Fi had described her daughter as 'depressed', but I was careful not to collude with the self-diagnosis; I wanted to explore what it meant for Maeve and Fi. I began by asking Maeve.

'I've noticed your mum has used the word "depressed" to describe what she's observed and I'm wondering what you make of that?'

'What do you mean?'

'Well, can you see why your mum thinks you could be depressed?'

'Yes.'

'Can you say more about that?'

'No.'

'That's okay… Could say what you think depressed means for you? It's not a test, by the way; it's just that the word can mean different things for different people, and I'm wondering what it means for you.'

Maeve shook her head; she either could not or would not elaborate, so I put the question to her mother instead.

'What about you, Fi? Can you say what depressed means to you?'

'Well, she's just so sad all the time. She cries a lot. She never goes out.'

'That's what you've observed in Maeve?'
'Yes.'
'What about depression generally? How would you describe that?'

I wanted to take the spotlight off Maeve for a bit as I could sense that she was finding it uncomfortable. I thought that some more generalised discussion might help.

'Well, if someone withdraws, spends a lot of time on their own, is never happy…'

'Are there any other things you think we might notice about someone who's depressed?' I asked this, not because I was testing Fi's knowledge about the characteristics of mental illness, but because I had a hunch that she might be worried about something else.

'Well, the really depressed ones might self-harm or do something stupid, you know?'

I thought I did know, but I needed her to say the words out loud, so that Maeve could hear what she was thinking too, and so I asked, 'Something stupid? Would you be able to say what you mean by that?'

'Kill themselves.'

'Yes,' I said, 'That can happen too.' I glanced at Maeve, who was shrunk uncomfortably in her chair and had started to cry.

'Is that a worry for you, Fi, that something like that could happen to Maeve?'

'Yes. I worry about it all the time. My biggest fear is that I'll come home from work one day and she'll be dead.'

I turned to Maeve and let her know that I had acknowledged her distress. 'I can see you're upset, Maeve. It is really upsetting to hear your mum say that she worries you could kill yourself.'

Maeve nodded but didn't say anything. I don't think she had the words. I wondered to myself what exactly was upsetting her – the knowledge that her mum was worried she could kill herself, or her own feelings that she might want to, or might try.

The reason I encouraged Fi to voice her concerns was to ensure that I had understood them, and, if Maeve was depressed or having suicidal thoughts, I needed to think about risk. I also wanted Maeve to hear how her mother truly felt – not to make her feel worse, which of course she might, but so that she knew that she mattered to her. Often when I speak to people who have thoughts of suicide, they are unaware, or have forgotten or need to be reminded, that they matter. They say things like, 'People would be better off without me.' I wanted

Maeve to know that her mother would not be better off, she'd be devastated. I continued my line of enquiry.

'I know it's hard, Maeve, but can you tell me if you have ever felt like you wanted to die?'

'Only every day,' she muttered.

'That's really sad to hear,' I said, because it was. It always is. I checked, 'And have you ever acted on those feelings? Have you ever done anything to try to end your life?'

'I've thought about it,' she answered.

Fi looked tearful now too and I asked her, 'Did you know that, Fi?' She shook her head.

'I think maybe at some level you did know, and that's why you've been so worried. Your instincts as Maeve's mum seem spot on.'

She nodded, so I continued to feed back what I thought I'd heard.

'I think what Maeve is telling us is that, while she has felt so sad that she has wanted to die and she has given that some thought, she hasn't done anything to try to end her life. Is that right, Maeve?'

'Yes, that's how I feel. And no, I've never done anything.'

Fi seemed to relax, reassured that Maeve wasn't at immediate risk, which was reassuring to me too. But it was still important to acknowledge Maeve's thoughts and feelings about ending her life. They needed to be taken just as seriously as any actions, or inactions, by her mother and by me.

Is it depression?

I had thought that suicidal ideation was probably the biggest concern for Maeve, and we'd acknowledged it quite early on in the consultation so that it didn't become 'the elephant in the room'. The other 'biggie' that Fi had mentioned in the referral was her concern about Maeve's eating. I named this and asked if Fi could explain her worries.

'She never eats.'

'I do!' Maeve corrected her.

'Not much,' Fi countered.

'I eat enough,' Maeve insisted.

Fi shook her head. 'You really don't, Maeve. You don't eat breakfast…'

'I'm not hungry in the morning!' Maeve interrupted.

'Okay, but what about lunch? You've stopped having lunch at school, you refuse to take a packed lunch…'

'No one takes packed lunches,' Maeve interrupted again. 'I'm not a 10-year-old!'

'I know you're not 10, love.' Fi sounded exasperated. 'But you still need to eat lunch.'

'Do you eat lunch, Maeve?' I asked.

'Not when I'm at school,' she admitted, 'because there's never enough time.'

'You don't get a lunch break?' I asked, knowing, of course, that she did.

'Not really.'

Fi looked at me with an expression that said 'See what I'm dealing with?' – and I did. I've seen it before, countless times, and I'm sure I will see it again, countless times more. I was seeing a 16-year-old girl who was restricting her food intake, skipping meals and refusing to eat when she was at school.

'What about dinner?' I asked.

'I eat dinner,' Maeve said, satisfied we couldn't argue with that.

I noticed Fi's expression change and Maeve's did too as she asked, 'What's that face about, Mum?'

'I don't want to get into an argument about it with you here, but…'

'No, say it,' Maeve said.

'Yes, say it,' I encouraged.

'Well, you do eat dinner, yes, but if we're being totally honest about it, you don't exactly have a healthy diet, do you?'

'What are you now? A dietician?'

Fi wasn't a dietician, and nor am I, but she had decided from observing her daughter that there were issues around food, and I had decided from observing the discussion between them that she was probably right. It was also clear that this was a touchy subject and that, for now, we should move on.

'From what you've both told me today, it's clear that things are really difficult for you just now, Maeve. I wonder if you can you say when you started to feel like this?'

She said she wasn't sure.

'Okay, I'll ask a different question: can you remember a time when you didn't feel like you do now? A time when you felt happy, perhaps?'

'Not really.'

'What about you, Fi? From your perspective, has Maeve always seemed sad?'

'Not at all. She was a happy little girl. She's always been a bit of an introvert, I suppose, but she's always had friends and enjoyed going to school, haven't you, love?' Maeve nodded and her mother continued. 'Thinking about it now, I suppose I noticed a difference in Year 9.'

'Year 9 – so when Maeve was around 13 or 14?'

'Yes, I think so.'

'What did you notice?'

'Well, she just started spending more time in her room, became a bit sulky. I don't mean to be rude, love, but that's just how I saw it.'

'It's okay,' Maeve reassured her mum, and I noticed the warmth between them.

'Did that worry you, Fi?' I asked.

'Not at the time,' she replied. 'I just thought, here we go, the teenage years are here!'

'Of course,' I said. 'The teenage years change us in lots of ways and it's quite ordinary to want more privacy, especially from our parents.'

Fi looked pensive. 'I suppose so. But I do wonder now if I missed something.'

'I wonder what you think you might have missed?' I asked.

'I don't know. The warning signs. The signs that something was wrong...' she trailed off.

'Perhaps there were warning signs, perhaps there weren't,' I offered. 'The other thing I'm wondering about is how much of what you noticed happening was ordinary, adolescent stuff, and how much of it was something else, something more worrying.'

Weighing up the ordinary against the worrying is always a consideration in my work, especially with adolescents.

'Depression, you mean?' Fi asked, reminding me that this was her main reason for contacting me.

'Possibly,' I said, 'but I'm more interested in trying to understand about Maeve's thoughts and feelings, what they are about and where they might have come from, and less interested in labelling them. Does that make sense to you both?'

They said that it did.

I have strong feelings about diagnostic labelling, and I don't hide them. On the whole, I see it as less beneficial than psychological assessment and formulation as a tool for understanding young people. However, more than two decades in child and adolescent mental health means that I have a good understanding of the diagnostic criteria for a range of conditions and disorders, and I cannot unknow what I know, or ignore those characteristics when I see them. I say 'characteristics', rather than 'symptoms', intentionally, so as not to medicalise the thoughts, feelings and behaviours that young people display. What I'd heard about Maeve was social withdrawal, school refusal, a poor relationship with food, low mood and prolonged suicidal ideation. According to the diagnostic criteria, these did indeed point towards depression (NHS, 2019). However, labelling it as such would, in my view, shut down any further exploration about what was going on and would be unlikely to change anything. I had a hunch that there was something else that could be relevant and I was curious to work with Maeve to find out what that might be.

Left behind

Maeve attended individual sessions of psychotherapy for about six months, reporting each week that she felt 'the same', which meant she was still sad, still withdrawn, still not attending school very often and still finding it difficult to engage when she did. I checked in with her regularly about suicidal thoughts and feelings, and she reported fluctuations. Some nights she cried herself to sleep, wishing she was dead. Some days she woke up relieved to be alive. Some weeks she reported not having thought about dying for a few days. So, by checking in with Maeve and asking the difficult questions directly – 'Have you thought about killing yourself this week?', 'Have you had any suicidal feelings since I last saw you?' – we were able to establish that her feelings weren't 'the same' but that they changed. The changes were only subtle, perhaps, but she had bad days and better days, and she began to see these fluctuations as being quite ordinary. Maeve never reported any motivation or intent to kill herself, and I shared this feedback with Fi during our therapy review meetings, every six weeks or so.

Maeve and I attempted to trace the origins of her difficult thoughts and feelings, and we worked out that she started to be aware of feeling 'like this' towards the end of Year 8, which was also the year she started her periods and had her first boyfriend. I was curious about this and asked if she could tell me more.

She said of her boyfriend, 'We were a perfect match, so when he asked me to be his girlfriend, I said yes.'

'Did you like him?'

'Not especially.'
'But you agreed to be his girlfriend?'
'Yes.'
'I'm curious about that…'
'All the other girls had had boyfriends already, but I hadn't.'
'So, you felt left out? Left behind, perhaps?'
'I'm always the girl that's left behind.'
'In what way?'
'Just that everyone else always has things first or does things first, before me.'
'What kind of things?'
'Everything! I was the last one to get a phone, the last one to be allowed to walk to school on my own. Everyone started their periods and got boobs before I did, not that I've got much now, and they all had boyfriends before I did.'
'I think I remember you telling me that you started your periods and had your first boyfriend towards the end of Year 8.'
'The boyfriend was in Year 8. My first period came that summer, before I started Year 9.'
'So, you were 12 or 13?' I checked.
'Yes, 12 when I had my first boyfriend and just turned 13 when I got my period.'
'I don't think that's especially late.'
'Don't you?'
'No, I think it's about average.'
'Oh, God, average is even worse than late!'
'Is it?'
'Yes. Average is so… I don't know… *average!*'
We both smiled.

I was interested in what Maeve had said about being the girl who was always left behind. Even if that wasn't true, it was how she felt, so it was true for her, and it had become a fixed, internal narrative. I knew that Maeve's birthday was in late August, so she would have turned 13 in the summer between Year 8 and Year 9, meaning that she was younger than most of her year group. In the UK, children start school in the September after their fourth birthday. So, for Maeve, this was a matter of days later, while someone born in September starts school the following September, a year later, when they are almost five.

A year can make a big difference when we are little. We think about development in terms of milestones, such as weaning (around 6–12 months), walking (around 12 months) and talking in short sentences (around 12–18 months). This way of tracking development according to chronological age continues throughout childhood. We expect most two-year-olds to be able to imitate adult behaviour in their play, identify pictures in a book and respond to simple instructions. By the age of three, we expect them to demonstrate an awareness of time, maintain a longer attention span and ask lots of questions – like, why, why, *WHY*? Between the ages of four and five, cognitive ability moves on apace, so that by the time children start school, assuming they start school at five, most will be able to count, draw and narrate pictures, name and identify colours, speak in longer sentences and recognise rhyming words (Very Well Mind, 2019).

In the UK, testing children starts young, with the first Standard Assessment Tests (SATs) to measure ability in maths and English in Year 2 and a second set in Year 6. Fast-forward five years and young people in the UK face their biggest tests yet in the form of GCSEs. So, throughout their school careers, children and young people face a lot of expectations, which are all based on the assumed age of their academic year group. Is that fair? Does it put summer-born babies (who do SATs aged six and 10, and GCSEs aged 15) at a disadvantage compared with autumn, winter and spring-born babies (who do SATs aged seven and 11, and GCSEs aged 16)? There is some evidence to suggest that August-born children get lower exam results, are more likely to leave education early, are less likely to get into a high-performing university, and are more likely to feel unhappy and to be diagnosed with ADHD (Whiteley et al., 2018). I wonder if that means that young people like Maeve are predisposed to be – or feel like they are – left behind, purely as a result of their birthday and arbitrary test dates, and whether they are inclined to feel as if they are always playing catch up. It seemed to me that, for adolescents like Maeve, a year could make a big difference.

I recalled that Maeve had described her first boyfriend as her 'perfect match' and I wondered if that was because he also felt left behind.

She said, 'No, it's because he was fat and ugly.'

I was taken aback. 'And you thought that was a perfect match for you because…'

'Because I was fat and ugly too. Because I *am* fat and ugly.'

'I'm surprised to hear you describe yourself in that way, Maeve, because I don't see you as fat *or* ugly.'

She lowered her eyes and seemed embarrassed or ashamed. What I thought didn't matter, in a way, but I said it to make it clear that how Maeve *felt* about how she looked bore little resemblance to how she *actually* looked; the fantasy didn't match the reality.

'I'm sorry to hear you describe yourself in that way. I wonder if you've felt like that for a long time.'

'I have.'

'Can you say how long?'

She shook her head.

'Okay. Can you think of a time when you didn't think you were fat and ugly?'

'I can't remember thinking differently about myself at the time, but when I look at old photos, I think I looked okay. Better than I do now, anyway.'

'When you say old photos, can you say how old? Do you think you looked okay at four or five, when you started school?'

'Yes, I think I was quite cute then.' She smiled and I smiled too.

'What about at seven, eight or nine, during primary school.'

'I think I looked okay then, too.'

'And what about at 10 or 11, when you were leaving primary and starting secondary school?'

'Mmmm… I'm not sure.'

'Twelve or 13.'

'I was definitely fat and ugly then. I think that's when I noticed it.'

'So, you started to feel differently, more negatively, about the way you looked around the time you were becoming a teenager?'

'Yes, I suppose so.'

'Around Year 8 into Year 9?'

'Yes.'

'The time you started your periods and got your first boyfriend?'

Maeve nodded.

'I'm also remembering what your mum said she noticed around that time. She thought you were a bit withdrawn and began spending more time in your room.'

'Yes, I think that all happened around the same time.'

'I'm wondering if those things might be linked.'

'I'm wondering too,' she said. 'I haven't thought about it before.'
'I'm also wondering what else might have been going on around that time, Year 8 into Year 9.'
'That's when I stopped eating.'
This was an important disclosure, and I was grateful that Maeve felt able to trust me with it. I encouraged her to continue.
'You stopped eating?'
'Yes. I stopped eating breakfast and I used to try and hide my school lunch. I told my mum I wanted to stop taking packed lunches and have the money to buy something instead...'
'Because it's easier to hide money, or spend it on something else, than it is to hide a packed lunch.'
'Yes, that.'
'Do you know why you started restricting what you ate?'
'Because I was fat.'
'And you wanted to lose weight?'
'Yes.'
'And again, I'm remembering what we talked about with your mum, and her saying that she's worried about your eating now. Do you understand why she's worried?'
'I suppose so.'
'Are you worried?'
'A bit. It's weird. I know it's bad not to eat, but not eating makes me feel better, in a way.'
'Better how? And I don't think it's bad or weird, by the way.' I tried to reassure her that I wasn't judging her eating behaviour; I was trying to make sense of it.
'Well, if I feel my stomach rumbling because I've not eaten, then I feel good about myself, that I've achieved something, you know?'
'Yes, I think I understand what you're saying. You want to feel as if you have some control over what happens to your body and how your body feels.'
'Yes, that's right.'

Food for thought

Working with 16-year-old girls, in particular, the theme of eating, or not eating, is a common one. Sometimes it relates to body image, as seemed to be the case for Maeve; sometimes it's linked to trauma, neglect or abuse, and other times the origins are less clear. But frequently an adolescent's relationship with food says a lot about their relationship to their sense of self and to their developing body. I wondered if, for Maeve, there was a link between not eating and wanting to remain younger and pre-pubescent – probably not consciously, but perhaps at some deeper psychological level. Being young, or 'left behind', felt familiar to Maeve, even though it wasn't a nice feeling. But she had a 'nicer' self-image in her pre-teen years than she did once puberty wreaked its hormonal havoc, and so it would make sense to want to maintain, or return to, that nicer feeling about herself, which she associated with an earlier time in her life. Adolescence is also the developmental stage when our bodies undergo a significant amount of change, when we may want to try to regain a sense of control over them by experimenting with clothes, hair, make-up, exercise and sex, as well as what (or who) we put into them.

It is important to note that, while Maeve's eating was clearly disordered, she did not present as someone with an eating disorder. She was a healthy weight for her age and size, and I discovered that, as well as days when she restricted her eating, there were days when she 'ate loads', and others when she 'ate normally'. These self-reports were reminiscent of the way Maeve had spoken about suicidal thoughts and feelings – that is to say, there were fluctuations in her eating patterns, with bad days and better days and days when it wasn't an issue at all.

If she had presented as unwell and I had suspected an eating disorder, my course of action would have been different and would have included her parents and possibly specialist services, in line with my contract, in which I state that, if I am worried about a young person's immediate safety, we may have to talk to someone else about that together because it wouldn't be fair on the young person to keep it to ourselves. Eating disorders (like suicidal ideation) pose a level of risk and, in the worst-case scenarios, a risk of death. But disordered eating (as opposed to an eating disorder) and thoughts of death (as opposed to suicidal intent) are not uncommon during adolescence, as young people work out who they are in relation to their mind, their body and the world. The period of adolescence is risky *per se*, due to the influence of sex hormones, which, as well as preparing us for adulthood, trigger impulsive and uncontrollable behaviour. The main causes of death during adolescence – drug use, traffic accidents and suicide – happen as a result of impulsive behaviour (O'Keane, 2021).

It is not uncommon for adolescents to think (and speak) in all-or-nothing kinds of ways – what is commonly called 'black-and-white' thinking: 'I stopped eating' – 'I wanted to die' – 'Everybody had one except me'. It is important to acknowledge the unbearableness of the feelings inherent in those statements, rather than dismiss them as exaggerations or attempt to minimise them, which would have the effect of dismissing and/or minimising the feelings. Some nights Maeve cried herself to sleep, wishing she was dead, and sometimes she skipped meals. Some days she woke up relieved that she was alive, and some days she ate loads. Some weeks she reported not having thought about dying for a few days, and sometimes she ate normally.

All-or-nothing thinking is apparent in the ways that adolescents compare themselves with other adolescents too. Maeve's pronouncements that 'everyone had started their periods' and 'everyone had boyfriends' and 'everyone had boobs' were communications about the way she perceived herself in comparison with her peers, and were also acknowledgements of her search for recognition as a mature young woman. It's interesting that these comparisons were based around sexuality – menstruation, breast development and getting a boyfriend. As the psychoanalyst Susie Orbach says in her book *Bodies*, 'girls want to be seen, [and] to pass the threshold of physical attraction', and they look to their peer group for clues about where, if and how they fit in. But there's also a paradox, because they need 'to know they are special and individual, while existing as part of a peer group' (Orbach, 2009, p.120). As Maeve had said to me, average is even worse than late. This illustrates a classic adolescent dilemma between wanting to fit in/be the same as their peers and wanting to be noticed and recognised as an individual. Working with 16-year-olds poses a similar dilemma between normalising the feelings as an ordinary part of adolescent development and exploring the nuanced meaning for the individual in the room.

Is it body dysmorphia?

At the point of referral, the concerns for Maeve included social withdrawal, school refusal, a poor relationship with food, low mood and suicidal ideation. I was reluctant to label this set of characteristics as depression, even though it could be said to fit the criteria, and instead remained curious about what was going on for Maeve, while keeping a very close eye on risk. Thanks to her honesty and willingness to trust in the therapeutic process, I discovered she also had some anxiety related to her appearance, and I wondered if this was what was fuelling her behaviour. I noted her self-description as 'fat and ugly' (which she was not) and put it into the context of her avoidance of social situations and school, her restricted eating and her suicidal ideation. Another potential diagnosis came to mind: body dysmorphic disorder (BDD), a condition characterised by a preoccupation with perceived defects or flaws in appearance that are not apparent to others (NHS, 2020).

The onset of BDD can often be traced to the onset of puberty (usually 12–14 years) and its features can become more apparent in late adolescence (16–18 years). Maeve ticked lots of BDD boxes: the way she felt about her appearance affected her mood, her school and social life, her relationship with food and her behaviour (National and Specialist OCD, BDD and Related Disorders Service for Young People, Maudsley Hospital, 2019). She started to notice difficulties around the age of 12 or 13, and these feelings escalated during her middle teens. But, while she was distressed by her perceptions of her appearance, her behaviour did not seem pathological. Again, as with the query about depression, I didn't think a diagnosis would serve much purpose for Maeve. That said, I added it to my mental list of things to keep a close eye on in terms of assessing and monitoring risk.

I reflected on the apparent need to label Maeve's behaviour – as depression, and/or an eating disorder, and/or BDD – and wondered whose need that was. It had been her mother, Fi, who had first brought it up at our initial consultation, but it had remained at the back of my mind throughout our work. My understanding of this was that it symbolised a need *for all of us* to make sense of Maeve's behaviour: 'Why is she behaving/thinking/feeling like that?' – 'Oh, it's because she's depressed/has an eating disorder/has BDD.' A label, on the face of it, can seem like a neat way of doing that. But a label doesn't make sense of the complexities of the individual adolescent's mind, or their feelings or behaviour, in the way that a therapeutic relationship can, as Maeve was discovering.

Loving and being loved

It will be of little surprise to hear that people with low self-esteem, high levels of self-criticism and a sense of inadequacy find it difficult to form and maintain healthy relationships. According to psychoanalytic literature, reparation of the internal world is needed to bring about identification with a loved object, rather than identification with a damaged and hated one (G. Williams, 1997). Another, more quaint and less analytical way of saying this is: we need to learn to love ourselves before we can love others or accept their love. Maeve had developed an internalised sense of herself as 'fat and ugly' (damaged and hated), which meant that she identified with those people who she perceived as 'fat and ugly' (damaged and hated) too.

Sometimes this sense of self comes from an experience of childhood adversity, such as trauma, neglect or abuse. As the psychotherapist Laurie Kahn says in her book *Baffled by Love*, 'Love is why they come to therapy. Love is what they want…' (Kahn, 2017, p.xiii). I think this could be said of anyone who comes to therapy, not just those with adverse childhood experiences (ACEs). And I think that identification with a damaged and hated object can also be a more generalised experience. The therapeutic encounter offers an experience of being nurtured and cherished that is quite unlike any other. It gives young people like Maeve an opportunity to get to know (and love) themselves, and to be known (and loved) by someone else, slowly, gradually and according to no one's timescales but their own. By slowing things down, paradoxically, it allows them to move on, to become unstuck, and to stop being 'left behind' in their old ways of thinking, feeling and behaving. It can help them to grow and to grow up.

Maeve had apparently begun to experience what could loosely be described as mental health difficulties 'for no apparent reason'. I didn't buy it. The reason that became apparent to us was the onset of adolescence. I think that she developed issues around food and began to restrict her eating as a response to the physiological changes and sensations that occurred as her body started to transition from that of a girl to that of a young woman. These changes were beyond her control, so she replaced them with physical sensations that she *could* control. I think she withdrew and spent more time in her room as a way to avoid the envy, rivalry and comparisons that are ubiquitous among 16-year-old girls. By remaining the girl who was left behind – at home, out of school – she could (unconsciously and/or symbolically) duck out of the competition. I'd noticed that the comparisons she made between herself and her peers were based around female sexuality – menstruation, breast development and getting a boyfriend – not so much because she was in search of sex (not consciously, anyway), but because she was in search of greater self-esteem, and because sexuality is what adolescents use to try to get it (Orbach, 2009). She didn't want to be average, (who does?); she wanted to be better (don't we all?). And because she didn't feel that she was better, or even as good as, she sometimes felt like she wanted to take the ultimate way out, by being dead.

During the time I spent getting to know Maeve, I was impressed by her capacity to think and be curious – a capacity that seemed to be limited at the beginning of her therapeutic journey and that developed over time, in part as a result of the thinking and curiosity I modelled about her, to her. I didn't try to change Maeve; I simply wanted to get to know her. Something resonated for me in Gloria Steinem's book *The Truth Will Set You Free, But First It Will Piss You Off!* (which, by the way, might also be an apt description of therapy!): 'If we arrive as a petunia in a garden of roses and lilies, we probably will need… someone who knows a petunia when she sees one and helps us to bloom as ourselves' (Steinem, 2019, p.3). To borrow from that imagery, I think that Maeve had felt like a petunia in a garden of roses and lilies since around the age of 12 or 13. Her experience in therapy had, to continue the garden symbolism, enriched the soil of self-acceptance and enabled her to flourish *as a petunia*.

7

Mother and son

Gabe is displaying antisocial behaviour and has been accused of crime. He's got himself caught up with a gang and may be involved in dealing drugs. His mother worships him. Can therapy help him to work it all out?

. . . .

Gabe was referred to me by a social worker who had been assigned to help his family. He had been referred to social care services by the local fire-setting team, who had received a referral from the police: Gabe had been among a group of boys and young men who had been caught setting fires in fields behind a housing development site. Members of the same group had been identified on CCTV, climbing into the back gardens of houses on nearby streets and breaking into garages. They were also thought to be involved in 'county lines' activity (the term refers to the mobile phone lines used by organised gang networks to make drug deals between one local authority and police jurisdiction (usually a big city) and another (usually smaller, more rural area)).

I remember thinking that Gabe had been around the houses, literally and metaphorically, to get to me – from the police to the fire-setting team, the fire-setting team to social care, social care to psychotherapy – which meant that his name was on a lot of reports, in a lot of files, in a lot of services. I was sent copies of several reports, along with the psychotherapy referral. I glanced over a couple and they made for grim reading. At best, they painted a picture of a reckless, helpless delinquent. At worst, Gabe was described as a demon, who went about terrorising the neighbourhood as part of a homogeneous gang.

I had heard about a spate of low-level crime (break-ins of garages and garden and allotment sheds) and anti-social behaviour (young people drinking in the streets, playing loud music and being 'intimidating') in the local news. I also knew about county lines. I wondered if Gabe was one of *those* characters in *those* news stories. I wondered too, what I might be getting myself into if I accepted the referral into my private practice, with no team around me to liaise with and share the load, and just monthly supervision for support. Would I become caught up in challenging unlawful behaviour? Would I be facing onerous ethical and safeguarding decision-making on a session-by-session basis? Would I be able to manage it/him?

I realised soon enough that, in considering the referral, I'd been heavily focused on thinking about risk – and mostly the risk to me, as a lone psychotherapist in private practice. At first, I felt ashamed for thinking about my own needs rather than Gabe's. But then I realised that maybe I *had* been thinking about Gabe's needs, which had been disguised as my own by my unconscious mind, in a countertransference reaction to the story I'd been presented with. To put it another way, in reflecting on what it would be like for me to work with Gabe without a 'gang' of my own who would 'have my back', had I inadvertently been wondering what it would be like for Gabe to be without a gang who had his? And was I wondering too about the dilemmas he might be facing on a day-to-day basis to do with risk and law-breaking, ethics and safety, and gang membership?

In asking myself whether I would be able to manage him, was I also wondering whether and how Gabe managed? I had lots of questions, but I also had one important answer – I accepted the referral and contacted Gabe's family to invite them to an initial consultation.

Conception and birth

I met Gabe with his mother, Gina. He was a tall, well-built, casually dressed young man, with shoulder-length blond hair and what struck me as a rather vacant expression. She was a small, fragile-looking woman in her mid-30s, who looked older. The thought passed through my mind that she looked as if she'd had a hard life. I soon learnt that she had. After making our introductions, I outlined the purpose of our meeting. Gabe said, 'She can talk,' gesturing with a tilt of his head towards his mother, who was seated next to him. His reticence to do the talking seemed like ordinary, understandable awkwardness about being put under the spotlight. He was probably aware that I had been made aware that he'd been under the professional spotlight plenty of times before.

My aim in an initial consultation is to learn about the current concerns for a young person in the context of their family background. Usually, I have lots of questions, but I didn't want to be cast in the same light as the slew of professionals who'd 'interrogated' Gabe previously. I wanted our first meeting, like any subsequent ones, to feel therapeutic. Ordinarily, I begin by asking about what's going on now and the cause for concern that has brought the family to therapy – the 'presenting issue', as therapists might call it. Then we work backwards, through the family and developmental history, all the way back to conception and birth. When I met Gabe and Gina, something told me to do it the other way around: to start with the parental relationship and work forwards to the present day. Gina seemed happy to talk and Gabe seemed comfortable enough to listen, so that's what we did, with them attending together over a number of weeks, because Gabe didn't want to come on his own.

I learnt that Gina and Gabe's father, Carl, had grown up in the same town, where their families had always lived and where Gina and Gabe still lived now. Carl was a couple of years older than Gina and had been friends with her cousin at school, so she was aware of him, but they only got together when she was 18 and he was almost 21. When I wondered what had attracted Gina to Carl, she said he made her feel safe, which I found interesting: it raised several questions – which I didn't voice, but mentally noted – about why she needed someone to make her feel safe; whether she had felt unsafe before she met him, and if so, why. Gina described Carl as 'a bit of a lad's lad', and when I invited her to elaborate, she said, 'He was well known, you know, always went around with a group of lads who everyone knew and everyone knew not to mess with.'

'Mess with how?' I wondered.

'Mess with at all! They were tough nuts, you know, a bit handy.'

'Handy?'

'Yeah. They knew how to look after themselves.'

'Oh, I see.' I sort of did. 'And they looked after you too?'

'Yeah, Carl did, and his mates, they were really protective.'

'That's how they made you feel safe?'

'Yeah. I felt like I was part of something, you know. Like part of this little gang that would always have my back. Not like gangs nowadays. More like a family, I suppose.' I noticed the steer away from 'gangs nowadays' – the kind of gang Gabe was allegedly involved in – but decided to stay with the theme of family.

'What about your own family, where were they?'

'Oh, they were here, but I mostly did my own thing.'

'You weren't close to your family?'

'Erm, it's hard to say. We were physically close, I suppose, but…' she trailed off.

'But maybe not so close emotionally?' I pondered.

'No, not emotionally.'

It felt like we were straying into Gina's stuff, which was interesting and relevant to an extent, because her stuff was Gabe's stuff too. As Fraiberg states at the very start of her groundbreaking paper, 'In Every Nursery there are Ghosts' (Fraiberg et al., 1975), meaning that parents unconsciously bring their own experiences of being parented into their relationships with their children. But I didn't want us to stray too far away from what was more clearly related to Gabe in our first meeting, and so I re-focused the discussion.

'So, you met Carl when you were 18…'

'Yeah.'

'And how soon did it become serious?'

'Very soon!'

'Okay, go on…' I encouraged.

'Well, I would stay over most nights, at his mum's place, and then I just stopped going home. Within the year I was pregnant with this little man.' She rubbed the top of Gabe's head and ruffled his hair like you might a much younger child.

'Mum!' Gabe moaned, but affectionately, as he pulled away.

'How was that, to find out you were pregnant, at, what… 19?'

'I was over the moon. So was Carl.'

'Great. So even though the pregnancy wasn't planned, it was a happy accident?'

'Yes, very happy.'

'And how was the pregnancy?'

'Fine. I had some sickness and a couple of scares, you know, but it was fine.'

'What kind of scares?'

'Pain mostly. Some bleeding.'

'That must have been worrying,' I suggested, aware that she was minimising the scariness of the 'scares'.

'It was a bit.'

'What support did you have?'

'Carl's mum was great. She went with me to most of the appointments.'

'And Carl?'

Gina grunted.

'What does that mean?' I asked.

'He didn't really get involved with the pregnancy. He said it was "girl stuff".'

'Even though he'd been *very* involved at the start?'

'Oh yeah, he liked *that* part!'

'I don't need to hear this, Mum!' Gabe interjected.

'No, son, I don't suppose you do,' she conceded.

We spared Gabe's blushes by moving away from discussing his parent's sexual history. I learnt that, after the birth, which, Gina said, 'looking back, was a bit traumatic', she and Carl and baby Gabe remained living at Carl's mum's house, along with his siblings and sometimes their boyfriends and girlfriends. It sounded like a busy household, with lots of people, all adults, coming and going. I tried to imagine what that must have been like for a new mother, not yet 20, with a new baby, living apart from her own family. Gina said she 'loved being a mum' but admitted that her relationship with Carl became 'a bit strained'.

'A new baby changes a relationship,' I acknowledged.

'Carl used to say, "There's three of us in this relationship and I think you're in love with the other man more than me".'

'He saw Gabe as the other man?'

'Yeah. I think he was jealous.'

'Of your love for your baby?'

'Yeah.'

'That must have been tough.'

'For Carl, maybe. But from the minute Gabe was born, he was the only man for me. He was my priority.' Gina raised her arm as if she was going to ruffle Gabe's hair again, but then thought better of it.

'How did things change between you and Carl, after Gabe was born?'

'He was out a lot. He'd go out drinking or smoking and come home late, when I'd got the baby to sleep, stinking of beer and weed, crashing about the place and wanting sex.' She glanced at Gabe. 'I didn't want that for my baby.'

'Or for yourself, I expect?' I half stated, half enquired.

'No.'

'What was it like for you, in those early days and weeks and months?'

'It was hard. I'd seen it before with my own parents. They say you end up with someone like your dad, don't they?'

'Some people do say that, yes. And I agree that we can get drawn to people who seem familiar to us, without always realising it at the time' – Freud's 'repetition compulsion' again (Freud, 1920).

I asked Gina, 'Are you saying that Carl was like your dad?'

'I didn't think so, not at first. I would *never* have chosen someone like my dad.'

'I wonder why?' I asked. Gina looked pensive but didn't answer, so I asked Gabe how he would describe his maternal grandfather.

'He's a bastard.'

'Oi!' Gina nudged him.

'It's okay,' I reassured him. 'And your dad, how would you describe him?'

'He's a prick.'

I asked Gina if she agreed with Gabe's descriptions of his father and hers, and their similarities.

She nodded and said, 'They both have a mouth on them and they're both handy with their fists.'

'Are you saying they are aggressive?' I asked.

'Can be.'

'And violent?'

'You could say that.'

'Would *you* say that, Gina?'

Gina nodded, but was reluctant to verbalise her agreement.

'So, to go back to what Gabe said, the two most important men in your lives, present company excepted, are bastards and pricks?'

'He's got a point,' Gina conceded, 'But I wouldn't describe them as important.'

'Wouldn't you?' I asked.

'Once, maybe. But not any more. This one's the only important man in my life. Has been for a long time.'

Ghosts in the nursery

Gina certainly seemed to hold Gabe in high esteem, perhaps too high, I thought, as if she had idealised (and possibly idolised) him, created a fantasy version of an ideal (idol) man, that may or may not (probably not) equate to the real young man in her life. I already had my suspicions about why that might be, and I thought it might, in part, relate to the ghosts in the nursery whose presence I'd already sensed. The field of psychoanalysis has tried to work out why and how some parents' early experiences get replayed in the lives of their children. This doesn't happen in every parent–child relationship, but it happens quite frequently in families that present in psychotherapy, as I've already discussed.

One theory is that, while the events of the past (such as trauma, neglect or abuse) might be remembered, the memory of the feeling (such as shame, fear or abandonment) is often repressed because it is too painful to hold in mind (Fraiberg et al., 1975). In scenarios such as these, it is not uncommon for the parent with the repressed feeling memory to re-enact, in some way, those unremembered affective experiences in relation to their child. Gina said she would 'never have chosen someone like her father' because she could remember what it was like to witness his drunkenness and his verbal and physical violence. What she was saying, in effect, was, 'I didn't want my child to experience what I'd experienced as a child.' However, despite her best intentions, Gina did unwittingly choose a man to father her child who shared characteristics with her own father. And, as a mother, she suffered the same sort of physically and emotionally abusive experiences that her own mother had endured.

But history is not destiny, Gina was not *her* mother and Gabe was not *his* mother – or his father. Gina described her mother's 'shut up and put up' approach to her aggressive husband, which, she thought, was a way to avoid 'adding fuel to the fire'. But in an effort to alleviate further conflict, Gina's mother had, in effect, colluded with her father to maintain the status quo, meaning that the background to Gina's childhood was one of domestic abuse. She hadn't framed it as such before, but now she could see that this was how it was. These were the ghosts in Gina's infantile nursery, but what about the ghosts in Gabe's?

I think that Gina's feelings from her childhood – of fear, of being hypervigilant to her father's moods and levels of drinking, of learning to be seen and not heard so as not to rile her father or make demands on her mother – were suppressed out of conscious awareness, but not fully repressed into her unconscious. Something drew her to Carl in the first place – something that, I suspected, felt familiar. She described him as making her feel protected, as a man who was 'handy with his fists' might well do, so long as his aggression and violence was turned outwards, against an external aggressor (a violent father, perhaps, or other violent man).

This can explain why some people choose violent partner after violent partner after violent partner, and say, unfathomably to outsiders, that they make them feel safe. But unfortunately, perhaps inevitably, sooner or later the violence turns inwards towards them (or their children), and that's when safe starts to feel unsafe, which is when a partner might decide to fight back or flee. In some relationships, the pattern of violence and abuse is re-enacted ad infinitum, partner to partner, to the next partner and the next; or from parent to child, who grows up and repeats the pattern some more, either as perpetrator or victim, depending on which parent they have identified with. But with Gina, once the warning signs were louder and clearer, she recognised that she 'didn't want that for [her] baby', and she chose to break the cycle. That said, I think the pattern created by the ghosts of Gina's past still cast a shadow on Gabe's nursery wall.

Metaphor

I like the metaphor of ghosts in the nursery because it helps to make sense of those remnants of the past, recreated in the present, that I witness in families, time and time again. I find metaphors useful tools in general in psychotherapy, because they help me to think about, as well as with, the young people and families I meet, who will often use them too. Psychotherapists frequently think, speak or describe their work as being 'in the metaphor', and we rely heavily on symbolism and symbolic interpretation, which again are helpful techniques in the quest for understanding and making sense of what emerges in the room. What can be less helpful is when metaphor morphs into euphemism and meaning becomes murky or open to misinterpretation. Reflecting on Gina's narrative, I realised that she used metaphorical jargon to avoid saying difficult things.

Carl had been described as a 'lad's lad', he was a 'tough nut' who was 'a bit handy' and 'had a mouth on him'. Gabe described him as a 'prick' and his grandfather as a 'bastard'. On the face of it, these statements sounded innocuous enough, but they seemed to me like veiled attempts to minimise Carl's verbally aggressive (had a mouth on him) and violent (handy with his fists) behaviour. The *Urban Dictionary* definition of 'lad's lad' seemed to sum up my impression of Carl perfectly. It states, 'a pure lad's lad is a male who specialises in creating and distributing exquisite banter and is generally seen as a mad cunt. Most true lad's lads are young... because a lad's lad cannot show any signs of maturity throughout his laddish career... common behaviour of a lad's lad is lack of consideration towards the female sex'.[1]

Gina had intimated that Carl was sexually demanding and that he didn't get involved in the 'girl stuff' of pregnancy, birth or childcare, which, for her, had involved 'a couple of scares' and was 'a bit traumatic'. Post-birth, their relationship became 'a bit strained'. On reflection, I felt that Gina's use of metaphor was a type of defence. By avoiding naming things as they really were (violent, aggressive, scary and traumatic), she could protect herself from thinking about, and perhaps accepting, those realities. I was reminded of this comment from a book about organisational culture: 'Panic finds uneasy containment in a language rich in metaphor' (Van Buskirk & McGrath, 1999). Nineteen-year-old Gina must have been filled up with panic about what would happen to her and her baby, and whether her old ghosts would come back to haunt them. I was unsure whether 35-year-old Gina was still holding onto a 'fantasy' and how much 'reality' she was ready to accept.

False idols

Just as Gina had (unconsciously) chosen to perceive Carl as a different version of the man he really was (unlike/like her father), the same could be said of how she perceived Gabe (unlike/like his father). My sense was that the 'Gabe in her mind' – that is to say, the fantasy Gabe – was an idealised version of the reality. I was interested in Gabe's name and asked Gina, as I often ask families, how it was chosen and by whom. She said she wanted a name beginning with 'G' like hers, because her baby was a part of her. I noticed that there was no consideration of a name beginning with 'C' or of immortalising the fact that Gabe was part of Carl too. Maybe Carl's sense of being displaced as the most important man in Gina's life once Gabe was born had been justified? Gina told me that when she discovered she was having a boy, she searched the internet for a 'good, strong name' and thought that something with one syllable sounded 'solid'. So, as I'd suspected, the

---

1. Urbandictionary.com

name Gina chose for her baby was imbued with meaning, which had implications for the meaning she projected onto her son too. She had chosen a good, strong, solid name, for a good, strong, solid boy, who was a part of her.

Before this conversation, I'd wondered if Gabe was short for Gabriel (which in this case, it wasn't), and had pondered on the meaning of the traditional Hebrew name, 'God is my strong man', derived from 'strong man or hero' (*gever*) and 'God' (*el*).[2] Gina had acknowledged the strength of the name and had, in a way, described Gabe in quite heroic terms. Although she denied any religious beliefs or reasoning behind the choice of her son's name, its sacred significance still interested me, in light of what I'd learned about the mother/son relationship. Gabriel is described in Christian, Jewish and Islamic scriptures as not just an angel but an *archangel*. Gabe was described by Gina not just as a son but as 'the only important man in my life', which was quite an elevation. In religious texts, Gabriel is a heavenly messenger. I wondered about the message Gabe could give to Gina – or, in other words, what he could teach her. There also seemed to be a link, in my mind, between the heavenly, God-like versions of 'Gabriel' and the sense I had that Gina worshipped Gabe almost as an idol (or false idol).

We might think of these creative musings as fantasies, in that they didn't exist in reality for the family I was working with. But the fact that they existed in my mind at all, in relation to Gina and Gabe, was significant. I'd had these particular fantasies in relation to this particular family and so, I believed, they must bear some relevance to them. The question with therapists' fantasies about the people they're working with is what to do with them. If I'd started talking about Gabe's potential role as a heavenly messenger, or Gina's idolatry, or the ghosts in the nursery, they'd probably have thought I was mad and run for the door. But I don't think we can (or should) ignore our fantasies, because they can be thought of as messengers too. Fantasies develop from a combination of past experiences and information (external stimuli), as well as thoughts, feelings and instincts (inner stimuli) (Salzberger-Wittenberg, 1970). But fantasy can also be used as an immature form of psychological defence, along with projection, passive aggression and acting out (Vaillant, 1994). I wondered if that

---

2. behindthename.com

was where my unconscious was leading me, into an exploration of the defences that Gina and Gabe were using and the potential meaning that could be assigned to them.

In Christian teaching, idolatry is viewed as a sin, akin to worshipping other/false gods, rather than the one true God. Gabe was Gina's only son, but Gina was one of two parents. I wondered if, by idolising him, she was projecting her own need to be idolised as the one true (good) parent, while splitting off (unconsciously) Gabe's (bad) father? Splitting things or people into all good or all bad is also, like projection and fantasy, a form of defence. Furthermore, in idealising Gabe and setting him up as a sort of idol, as I suspected was the case, Gina could split off and therefore deny the less heroic, less idealised parts of her son, which she felt belonged to Carl. I'm not suggesting that Gina was aware of what her unconscious mind had been up to, because all this defensive sorting out happens – well – unconsciously, and, as Freud taught us, we are not responsible for the behaviour of our unconscious mind (Freud, 1909). However, now that I had become aware of what *my* mind had been thinking and fantasising about, I could bring some of that into the sessions with Gina and Gabe in a more conscious and (I hoped) palatable way.

The other side of the law

I asked Gabe how it felt to hear his mum describe him as the only important man in her life.

He said, 'It's a bit cringey. I wish she'd find herself a man of her own.'
'I don't need a man,' she declared, quick as a flash. 'I have you!'
'But you won't have me forever,' he asserted. 'I'll be gone soon.'
'Gone?' I asked. 'Gone where?'
'College, then uni, hopefully.'
'That's great,' I said. 'It's good to hear you have plans. What would you like to study?'
'I'm doing Health and Social at college. Then eventually I'd like to join the police.'
'Wow,' I said, remembering the reason for the referral, which so far had remained unmentioned, and wondering about the juxtaposition between being on one side of the law and wanting to be on the other.
'Are you on track?' I asked.
'Kind of.'
'What does "kind of" mean?'

'My predicted grades are sixes, maybe some sevens if I work hard, but my attendance hasn't been great this year.'

'How come?'

'Stuff going on, you know how it is…'

'I've heard from other people how *they* think it is. How do *you* think it is, Gabe?'

'It's not been that great, to be honest.'

'Thank you for your honesty. How come?'

Gina interjected, 'He's got himself mixed up with the wrong crowd.'

Another metaphor. 'What kind of wrong crowd?' I attempted to clarify.

'Some local lads who've been caught doing stuff they shouldn't.'

It sounded like she was describing a bunch of naughty little boys with their hands in the cookie jar, rather than a group of young adults who had been accused of fire-setting, vandalism, stealing and drug dealing.

'Okay,' I said, stalling for time, as I tried to decide whether to continue with this line of exploration or another. I opted for another. 'Has Gabe always found himself mixed up with the wrong crowd?'

'God, no. He was a good kid at primary school. Quite quiet, a bit shy, but always a good kid.'

'So, his recent behaviour is out of character?'

'Totally.'

'Is that how you saw yourself when you were younger, Gabe, as a good kid?'

'I suppose so. I just kept my head down and got on with it.'

'Did you have friends?'

'Yeah, a few.'

'What about a best friend?'

'Not really. There was always a group of us who lived on the estate. We'd ride to school together and hang out after school in the park.'

'Are you friends with the same group now?'

'Some.'

'They're toe rags!' Gina stated.

'Toe rags?' I asked.

'Yeah, you know, always up to no good.'

'Not all of them, Mum.'

'No, maybe not all of them. But you're better than that, Gabe. Better than them.'

'They sound like lad's lads,' I speculated, making a tentative link between Gabe's bunch of friends and Carl's.

'Exactly!' Gina agreed. 'And he's better than that,' she repeated.

'You seem to be saying that you want better for Gabe, that you don't want him to be like his dad,' I suggested.

'That's the last thing I want for him.'

'Do you see your dad, Gabe?' I asked, realising I only knew about Carl in the past.

'Not any more.'

'How come?'

Gabe looked to Gina, as if he was checking how to answer my question.

She said, 'He's inside.'

'In prison?' I clarified.

'Yeah. He got done for aggravated burglary. Not for the first time either.'

'I wonder what that's like for you, Gabe, that your dad's in prison?'

'Like I said, he's a prick.'

'You did say that, yes. But how does it feel for you that your dad's a prick who's in prison?'

'Ashamed.'

Gina was riled. 'You've no need to feel ashamed, Gabe, it's not you that's the prick!'

'It's not Gabe's fault, you're right. But I think his feelings are valid. It's a difficult thing to hold in mind the knowledge that your dad's in prison. I think I understand why Gabe might feel shame, and perhaps some anger and resentment too.' Gabe nodded.

'Maybe you worry that your dad's behaviour might affect you in some way, that you might be tarred with the same brush?' Now *I* was resorting to ambiguous metaphor!

'I hate people knowing.'

'Of course,' I reassured him. 'What's it like for you when they find out?'

'The kids on the estate, the "toe rags" as Mum calls them, think it's like a badge of honour.'

'A badge of honour for you that your dad's in prison?'

'Yeah.'

'Are their dads in prison too?'

'Some of them. One got sent down recently for possession.'

'Possession of drugs?' I checked.

'Yeah.'

'Badger's always been an arsehole,' Gina said, as if by way of explanation. 'I've never liked him.'

'You know Badger?' I asked.

'Yeah, he was one of Carl's mates, back in the day.'

'Yes of course,' I said. 'I'd forgotten that you all grew up together.'

'They were thick as thieves,' she said, with no pun intended.

'That's why I want out,' Gabe said.

'To get away from the past?' I asked.

'Yeah.'

'And to put yourself on the *other* side of the law to your dad?'

'Yeah, I hadn't thought of it like that before, but yeah, definitely.'

'I think your mum wants that for you too. And I think maybe that's what she wanted for herself.'

'What do you mean?' Gina asked.

'Well, I remember you saying that you didn't want to end up with a man like your father; you wanted your life, and your son's life, to be different to how your own childhood had been.'

'And look how that turned out!'

'Oh, I don't think it turned out so bad,' I reassured her. 'There were a few wrong turns along the way, perhaps, but you got Gabe, you got rid of Carl, Badger and the rest of them, you tried hard to do things differently...'

'I *have* tried hard,' she said, and then, to my surprise, and hers too, she broke down, as if she had finally become aware of all the feelings – from her childhood, her relationship, and her more recent past – properly and intensely, for the first time. 'Oh God, I'm sorry,' she sobbed. Gina's apology was directed at me for her tears, which I assured her was unnecessary, but it also seemed to be an apology to Gabe – *for everything.*

Back to reality

Before I met Gabe, I'd been set up by 'the system' to think of him as a juvenile delinquent. He'd been caught setting fires, caught on CCTV breaking and entering and caught up with a gang who were dealing drugs. As I got to know him and his mother, I began to perceive him as caught up in something else too, something not quite real, or something that didn't belong to the here and now, or that maybe didn't even belong to him. It was interesting that, without really planning it that way, I'd ended up 'doing therapy' with Gabe *and* Gina. I wondered if, unconsciously, he'd been set up to be referred on her behalf; as if he'd been the messenger, perhaps, or at least as if his behaviour had been. It happens sometimes, that the 'thing' that precipitates a referral to psychotherapy contains fragments of the past, and this can be the 'launching pad for change' (Byng-Hall, 1995, p.3). The 'thing' that triggered Gabe's referral was his antisocial and criminal behaviour. I knew that was true; I'd read about it in the reports, and he'd admitted it to me himself, but nevertheless, it didn't fit with my sense of him as a 'good kid' as opposed to a 'lad's lad'. It just didn't make sense, and we all desperately needed it to make sense if Gabe was to achieve his predicted grades, go to college and position himself on the right side of the law.

The antisocial and criminal behaviour I'd heard about could be described as 'acting out', which is an ordinary part of childhood development and which changes in how it manifests as children transition through different stages and grow in age. Acting out can look like tantrums in two-year-olds and sound like rageful cries of 'I hate you' in the teenage years. Throughout puberty, a common form of acting out is stealing. These are the ordinary ways that ordinary young people assert themselves, by staging a protest ('I'm not a child any more, I don't have to do what you tell me to do'), or a statement about their needs ('If you won't give it to me, or I perceive you as giving it to someone else in my place, I'll take it for myself in order to deprive someone else of it') (Waddell, 2018). Gabe's acting out had gone to the next level and seemed like more than ordinary, developmental stuff. I wondered if his kind of acting out was a defence (against what, I wasn't yet sure), but it seemed to have a different meaning, something he'd become caught up in unknowingly.

The gang

Another thing Gabe had become caught up in (in reality) was a gang. I wracked my brains for where I'd heard that before in our sessions and remembered Gina's descriptions of what it was like when she started going out with Carl. She said she felt 'part of this little gang' that protected her and made her feel safe. In writing about gang dynamics, it has been stated that, 'The gang gets together under the guise of offering protection to its members, but its primary task is to do damage' (G. Williams, 1997, p.53). I remembered my reflections, before meeting Gabe, about what it would be like for me, as a therapist in private practice, to work with a member of a gang, without a gang of my own. Who would protect me? I had hypothesised that this was a countertransference response in relation to considering what it would be like for Gabe to be without his gang. In her paper, 'From a Gang of Two', the psychotherapist Sue Kegerreis talks about the ways that siblings form a gang and suggests that gangs offer the comfort of a 'narcissistic relationship' as an alternative to the 'pain of dependence'. Furthermore, she implies that loyalty to the gang is demanded over any other relationship that might threaten it (Kegerreis, 1993).

I wondered now about the 'gang of two' that consisted of Gabe and Gina, who weren't siblings, of course, but Gina certainly seemed to have skewed the relationship (in her mind) into a horizontal, side-by-side, sibling or partner one, rather than a vertical, parent/child one. Gina described Gabe as 'the only man for me', which certainly intimated a level of loyalty towards their relationship above all others, and this seemed to be about her own (narcissistic?) needs and her own avoidance of becoming dependent on another man – who might turn out to be like Carl or like her father. Perhaps then, Gabe's acting out in a delinquent gang was a defence against becoming dependent on the gang of two. Perhaps it was his way of separating from his mother, by choosing a gang of his own. Perhaps it *was* a sign of ordinary adolescent developmental stuff, albeit gone slightly awry.

In his paper 'Delinquency as a Sign of Hope' (which I think is a reassuringly normalising title), Winnicott suggests that antisocial behaviour contains an SOS (Winnicott, 1986b). This SOS is a communication, a *message*, if you like, about what is going on for the so-called antisocial young person. According to Winnicott (and others), the behaviour can often be traced back to its origins in a parental break-up, which causes something to happen in the child's mental organisation – that is, in their mind – triggering aggressive thoughts and impulses. According to psychodynamic theory, the loss of a father, as was Gabe's experience, also raises (unconscious) Oedipal anxieties in the child and the fear that it is their own aggressive thoughts that have caused their father to be destroyed (Freud, 1910). When aggressive thoughts and impulses begin to feel threatening, they are acted outward, in an effort to get rid of them, as a form of defence. So, the message contained within the antisocial behaviour is, 'I don't feel safe'. And what better way is there to feel safe than to become part of a gang, with its 'guise of protection'? My deliberation on the meaning of gangs appeared to have taken me full circle.

Reflecting on why they came

I couldn't have predicted how my work with Gabe and Gina would pan out. It started with a referral to psychotherapy for a 16-year-old who'd been accused of setting fires, breaking into garages and sheds and dealing drugs. He'd been characterised as wicked and threatening, a sort of demon, a member of a gang. The young man I met was nothing like that. He was ambivalent, reticent and had lost his way on the road to adulthood. His ambivalence about engaging in therapy meant that his mum came too, and what started off as her accompanying him to his initial consultation and helping him to tell his story turned into her telling hers over several weeks, which we all came to realise was the prequel to his.

I often think that the parents of young people in therapy are courageous. Despite wondering (and/or worrying) about the family secrets that might be shared, or whether they will be portrayed in a good light, and what I might think of them and where that might lead, they allow their children to attend, and many even pay, sometimes for months or even years. What I think is even more courageous is a willingness to be part of the process too, either in parent–child or family work, to open up their own cans of worms and their own Pandora's boxes, as Gina did. She also opened up her mind to the reality that Gabe was a young man in his own right, not a man just for her. By sharing the secrets of her own childhood and relationship with Gabe's father, she had modelled thinking, processing, digesting and open-mindedness to her son in ways that a brave, thinking, loving, nurturing, good-enough parent can. Which was way more impactful for Gabe than anything I could have offered him in individual psychotherapy.

I am reminded of a quote (which I think belongs to the psychoanalyst Wilfred Bion) along the lines of, 'If you knew why, you would not be here; you would not have wasted time coming. You came here to see me precisely because you did not know why you had come.' I think it fits my work with Gina and Gabe perfectly: neither of them knew (consciously) why they came to therapy, but they worked it out.

8

Learning to live

Belle has been in hospital following another suicide attempt and her mother doesn't understand why her daughter wants to die. Can psychotherapeutic thinking untangle their narratives, so that Belle can choose to live?

. . . .

Emmy asked to consult with me about her daughter, Belle, who was at the time an inpatient in an adolescent psychiatric unit. Belle had disengaged from school, social life and everything in between and had been admitted to hospital following a 'serious suicide attempt' – Emmy's words, not mine. I think that all suicide attempts are serious. Belle was due to be discharged a few weeks later, and Emmy was hugely concerned, understandably, that, once home and away from the 24-hour care and scrutiny of the trained team of professionals, Belle might do it again, this time on Emmy's watch. I heard that Belle had attempted to end her own life several times before. She had taken numerous overdoses of over-the-counter (paracetamol and ibuprofen) and prescription (antidepressant and sleeping pills) medication. The first time, according to Emmy, was when she was about 12. I had a hunch that it might have been earlier, because parents often aren't aware of the first time.

I wondered what had gone on for Belle that she had felt so desperate, at such a young age, and asked Emmy if she had any thoughts about a potential trigger. At first, she said she couldn't think of anything, so I prompted further and asked what Belle was like at 12. Emmy smiled wistfully and said, 'Just a normal little girl.' On the face of it, this was an endearing statement, but it didn't tell me much about Belle. It did, though, tell me something about her mother and about the mother–daughter relationship. I wondered about the choice of words and their underlying meaning. People might use the phrase 'normal little girl' to describe someone of seven or eight, perhaps even nine, or at a push, 10, but I wasn't so sure that 12-year-olds are little girls any more. They are pubescent adolescents, pre-teens with developing bodies and the hormonal urges to match. I wondered if Emmy's statement contained a veiled attempt to undermine that reality; to deny that, at 12, Belle was maturing into sexual young woman.

And what about the prefix 'just'? I wouldn't want to be described as anything preceded by 'just'. I find it demeaning when people say, 'just a stay-at-home mum' or 'just a secretary' or 'just a carer'. Perhaps that simple statement, 'just a normal little girl' would turn out to be my first clue about what might be amiss. Whether that originated from Belle or was a projection from Emmy, or communicated something about the relationship between the two, I was still to discover. For starters, I encouraged Emmy to think with me about how Belle went from being 'just a normal little girl' to a psychiatric inpatient in only four years.

She said, 'I really don't know. I don't understand it myself.'

'Yes, it is hard to understand,' I agreed.

'I don't know why she'd do it.'

'Try to end her life?' I asked. It was important to name 'it' explicitly and avoid vagueness or euphemisms.

'Yes. I've given her everything,' Emmy said.

'I notice you said "I" rather than "we". Can I ask about Belle's dad?'

'We split up when she was little.'

I wondered if Emmy meant 12-year-old little or littler, so I asked, 'How little?'

'Maybe seven…'

'What was that like, for Belle, I mean?'

'Fine, I think. She just accepted it.'

There it was again; that seemingly innocuous word 'just'. In my experience, a parental break-up isn't ever little and the feelings it evokes in a child are never 'just' acceptance. There seemed to be something about the way Emmy thought about big things and growing-bigger people that made them littler, minimised them and reduced their significance. Except for the latest suicide attempt, which she thought of as serious. Good. I was relieved to hear it; it *was* serious. Some people, rather unhelpfully in my opinion, describe suicidal behaviour as a 'cry for help' or, more dismissively, 'attention seeking'. The notion of attention seeking came to my mind as I spoke to Emmy about Belle, but in a 'let's think about why she did that' way, rather than a disparaging or dismissive way. If someone (perhaps a mother) has a tendency to minimise major life changes (say, the break-up of a marriage, or the coming of age of a daughter, or that same daughter's heightening state of distress), then it might take a lot to get their attention. The ante might have to be notched up a level in order for them to notice that something's wrong, and a 'serious' suicide attempt would do exactly that. I am not suggesting that Belle, who I hadn't even met yet, was consciously attempting suicide to get Emmy's attention, but I thought there might be some communication of her need to be validated by her mother in the complicated mix, and once I was aware of that thought, I held it in mind as I made my initial hypotheses.

Developmental breakdown

According to psychodynamic theory, suicidal behaviour can be perceived as a communicative 'cry for help' (Fox & Hawton, 2004) or a more reactive 'cry of pain' (J. Williams, 1997). The cry of pain theory takes into account the factors that precipitate suicidal behaviour – the antecedents or triggers – which might be external events in the outside world or internal, mental pain and distress, or both. According to Williams, suicide is a reaction to feeling defeated by, or trapped in, an unescapable situation: the suicidal individual believes suicide to be their only way out. As an aside, non lethal self harm, on the contrary, is thought to express a belief in the potential for escape (or rescue). I wondered about the internal and/or external influences on Belle's suicidal behaviour, which, according to her mother's account, had begun to feel inescapable around the age of 12.

Despite my suspicion that the behaviour had probably started earlier, I considered the potential implication of it becoming apparent at 12. This is a significant age of development – or, more precisely perhaps, of developmental breakdown (Laufer & Laufer, 1995). Psychoanalytic theory suggests that disruptions in adolescent functioning, such as those exhibited by Belle in her mid-teens, are the result of developmental breakdown at puberty. The Laufers were prominent members of the British Institute of Psychoanalysis. Moses Laufer trained as an adolescent psychoanalyst with Anna Freud, while his wife Eglé had originally worked in obstetrics, where she developed an interest in the role of the mother–baby relationship. This evolved into a fascination with the development of girls in particular, and the influence of early attachment to the primary object (the mother) on the adolescent's sense of her maturing body. I'm interested in those things too. The Laufers combined the understanding gained from their different earlier careers in their work together at the Brent Adolescent Centre and their jointly written and hugely influential book, *Adolescence and Developmental Breakdown* (Laufer & Laufer, 1995). Reflecting on their clinical work in the book, they share their repeated experiences of being struck by patients who report that, 'everything was going well, more or less, until something happened suddenly... after which things were never the same again' (p.21). I hear statements like this a lot too – variations on, 'It came from nowhere.'

I reflected on what Emmy had told me about Belle. She had 'just accepted' that her parents had separated, when she was about seven. At 12, she was 'just a normal little girl' who had taken an overdose in an attempt to end her own life. At 16, she was admitted to an adolescent psychiatric hospital following a 'serious suicide attempt'. I hypothesised that these headlines contained just as much, if not more, of Emmy's narrative as they did of Belle's. And as it was Emmy seated in front of me, I decided to explore her story further, to set the scene for Belle's.

A mother's story

I asked Emmy how she would describe her own childhood, and was unsurprised by her response.

'Just, you know, normal.'

'Just normal?'

'Yes.'

'I wonder what you mean by just normal?'

'Just that, really, nothing unusual. There was me and my younger sister, and my mum and dad.'

'And the four of you were together throughout your childhood?'

'Yes, mostly.'

'Mostly?'

'Well, dad left when I was about 12.'

'How do you remember that time?'

'I'm not sure. What do you mean?'

'Well, I'm guessing that things changed after your dad left and I'm wondering *how* they changed for you.'

'They didn't change much at all, really. He wasn't around very much before they split up. He used to work a lot, long hours. He was an accountant with his own business, and he often worked at weekends too. I don't think we really noticed he was gone!'

There it was again, that tendency of Emmy's to minimise big events. Perhaps that's where it began, with her father leaving. Perhaps that was the 'until something happened' moment in Emmy's adolescent experience that the Laufers wrote about.

'I wonder how your father would feel to hear you say that you didn't notice he was gone?' I asked.

'I don't know. It sounds bad, doesn't it?'

'Not bad, necessarily. But it's interesting to me that something so significant as your dad leaving had such a seemingly insignificant impact on you.'

'Yes, I see what you mean.'

'What about your sister, do you think it affected her differently?'

'Well, she's younger than me, by five years, so she was probably affected even less than I was.'

I did the maths. 'So, she'd have been about seven when your parents split up?'

'Yes.'

'About the same age that Belle was when you and her dad separated?'

'Yes! I hadn't realised that before!'

'I wonder what you think about it now that you *have* realised?'

'It's a bit of a coincidence, isn't it?'

'Perhaps.' I'm not sure I believe in coincidence, but I do believe in the significance of repetition and so I encouraged Emmy to think about that too. 'But perhaps it's interesting to acknowledge that you have twice witnessed someone close to you experiencing dads leaving when they were seven – first your sister, and then your daughter.'

'Yes…' Emmy seemed reflective. 'Do you think that means something?'

Because she'd asked me directly, I decided to share my thinking directly too, but carefully, and in a way that opened up further exploration, rather than shut it down with a definitive answer. This was mostly because I didn't have one; I was merely playing with an idea.

'I think that your first experience, of seeing how your sister responded to her dad leaving, might have influenced your later experience of seeing how your daughter responded to a similar event.'

'Yes, I can see that.'

'But 12-year-old you didn't think things really changed that much, because that's how you saw it. Maybe that's how you thought your sister saw it too?'

'Yes. I don't think I had much empathy at that age!'

'Empathy's a tough call for most 12-year-olds!' I assured her.

We both smiled. We'd needed that reprieve to lighten the tension a bit before we continued on our journey into Emmy's history. I'd been given a pointer about seven-year-olds and 12-year-olds in the family narrative. Next, it was time to discover the meaning of being 16. I asked Emmy what came to mind when she thought of herself at that age, and this time her answer *did* surprise me.

'I left school, joined a band, and lost my virginity to the lead singer!'

'Wow. Very sex and rock 'n roll!'

'I know. No drugs though! His name was Dan. He was 18 and absolutely gorgeous.' She smiled at the memory. I smiled too and encouraged her to continue.

'Well, we got together. He was my first serious relationship. My first love, I suppose, and we were inseparable. Then two years later, I found out I was pregnant. I actually took the pregnancy test on my 18th birthday.'

'Gosh, how was that?'

'I couldn't believe it. I was in denial. I dressed up, as planned. Went out with my friends, as planned. Drank too much, as planned. I didn't tell a soul.'

'That's a big thing to keep to yourself.'

'Not as big as what happened next.'

'Which was?'

'I lost the pregnancy. It was horrendous. I didn't know if I wanted to keep it at first. I was so young, about to start uni. I had my whole life ahead of me, you know. But when that happened...'

'It was still a loss.'

'Yes.'

'Can you tell me what happened, Emmy?' I had a feeling she hadn't told this part of her story before and that it was important for her to have it witnessed.

'I was coming up for 12 weeks. I had a little bump, you know, but I was able to hide it, until I was sure about what I wanted to do. And then, one day, I was at home on my own. It was a Saturday. My mum had taken my sister somewhere, thank God – gymnastics, I think, and I had this excruciating pain, and then, whoosh…' she gestured something being expelled from her body. 'It was terrifying. I'd never seen so much blood, lumpy blood, and clots.'

'You must have been very frightened.'

'I was terrified. I knew what it meant. No more baby.'

'Do you remember how you felt about that?'

'I was sad. But also relieved. Does that sound awful?'

'Not at all. It's understandable that your feelings would be a mixture of fear, sadness and relief. What happened next?'

'I had a shower, put my clothes in the washing machine and went to bed. When my mum got home, I told her I had a bad period. It didn't feel like a total lie. And then I just carried on like normal.'

I echoed Emmy's words back to her, 'You just carried on like normal…'

'Yes. I say that a lot, don't I?'

I smiled, pleased that she was becoming aware of what I'd been aware of too. 'You do.'

'I wonder why…?'

'Do you want to know what I think, Emmy?' She nodded. 'I think that when something big happens – say, your dad leaving, or Belle's dad leaving, or finding out about and then losing the pregnancy, or about your daughter's overdose – your mind tries to protect you from the unbearableness of the situation by shrinking it down, making it smaller, making it into "just" this little thing that you can manage. Does that make sense to you?'

'Absolutely. Like a defence you mean?'

'Yes, like a defence.' I smiled again.

Defence mechanisms

The concept of defences, or psychological defence mechanisms, to use its full and proper title, is widely understood beyond the psychoanalytic profession. What Emmy was referring to was denial, which is the rejection of reality, or the carrying on as if the denied thing – the miscarriage, for example – hadn't happened. She also acknowledged her tendency to minimise (or repress) – that is, to squash down out of conscious awareness – those realities that were difficult to be aware of, such as 12-year-old Emmy's response (or her seven-year-old sister's response) to their dad leaving, or her daughter's suicide attempts. The theory of defence mechanisms is usually credited to Sigmund Freud, the father of psychoanalysis, but it was most thoroughly examined and elaborated by his daughter Anna (Freud, 1937).

Credits aside, the important thing that the Freuds observed about defence mechanisms was their function in distorting reality in order to reduce feelings of anxiety. Another important point to note is that all of us, mentally healthy or otherwise, rely on defence mechanisms at some time or another, to a greater or lesser extent, to protect us from feeling anxious. Like all coping strategies, reliance on them only becomes problematic – or, in extreme cases, pathological – when it interferes with everyday physical and mental functioning. The rest of the time, defence mechanisms serve an important function in protecting us and allowing us to get on with our ordinary, day-to-day life, largely unhindered by unbearable thoughts and feelings.

Talking things over with me had brought into conscious awareness those thoughts and feelings Emmy had tried not to think about or feel because they were too unbearable. But the most unbearable thing of all was the fear that she wouldn't be able to keep her daughter alive once she was discharged from hospital.

Monitoring suicide risk

I empathised with Emmy's position. The weight of responsibility for a life is a heavy one to bear. Belle wasn't my daughter, I hadn't even met her, but I felt that weight too. What reassured me (slightly) was that the weight was shared by the team at the adolescent unit where Belle was an inpatient, and would continue to be shared by the home treatment team after she was discharged. I knew that they would have been monitoring her, caring for her, treating her with talking therapy and possibly medication, and all the while assessing the risk she posed to herself. I knew that the decision to discharge her would be made jointly by a group of multidisciplinary professionals and would come with a carefully considered care plan that included recommended treatment and regular reviews.

A key component of Belle's care plan was psychotherapy, hence the referral to me. I've mentioned elsewhere that medical professionals, including hospital teams, use quantitative assessment and outcome measures, such as strengths and difficulties questionnaires (SDQs), anxiety self-reports (GAD-7) and depression scales (PHQ-9). I've also mentioned the reasons that I don't use them: they don't consider the nuances of the individual's needs and the nature of their lived experiences. However, there are exceptions to every rule, even my own, and this felt like an exceptional situation. I sensed that Emmy was at a loss. I knew she was asking herself, and me, 'How will I know if Belle's okay?'; 'How will I know if she's going to do something to hurt herself again?' and 'Will I be able to keep her safe?' Emmy needed to feel well enough resourced to support her daughter. She'd found me, and brought me on board to offer a space to think about the emotional burden of caring for Belle, but she also needed practical resources; she needed to feel she could *do* something.

I decided to suggest a simple assessment tool designed by the mother of a severely depressed adolescent that I remembered reading about in *Navigating Teenage Depression* (Parker & Eyers, 2010), a very accessible, common-sense book for parents and professionals. I gave Emmy a copy to read and referred her to the risk assessment questions:

- How bad (in all sorts of ways) are they?
- Are they 'themselves' or not?
- What impact is their mood state/behaviour having on their life?
- Are you worried about them not coping?

The authors suggest rating each question on a scale of 1–10, and I encouraged Emmy to set a threshold – that is, to ask herself, how high would the score need to be, and for how many of the questions, for her to be really worried. I also reiterated that, if she had any suspicion whatsoever that Belle had the intention, motivation or plan to end her life, she should contact a professional immediately – either the local accident and emergency department, the home treatment or crisis intervention team, or me. The sad fact is that, if someone is intent on ending their life, they probably will, but that doesn't mean that we shouldn't do what we can to safeguard them. That said, according to recent research, suicide accounts for only 1.4% of all deaths (Soper, 2018), which the researcher suggests is due to an innate human instinct to survive. Emmy was grateful for the book and thought the risk assessment tool might be helpful. We set a date for her to bring Belle to an introductory appointment with me the week after she was discharged from hospital.

Second skin

I met Belle for the first time, with her mother, on a warm summer's day, although her presentation belied the weather. She was dressed head to toe in black: a black, long-sleeved cardigan over a black, high-necked sweater, tucked into a woollen black mini skirt, over black opaque tights that disappeared into chunky black Doc Marten boots. Layer upon layer of heavy black protection. Belle's hair, however, was a vivid shade of purple, recently dyed (to my eyes), and styled to form perfect curls that framed her face and fell neatly to her shoulders. She wore expertly applied make-up that accentuated her eyes with black kohl and perfectly plucked eyebrows. Her lips were outlined and filled with a deep shade of red.

There seemed to me to be a mismatch between Belle's head and her body. A head and shoulders shot would show a young woman who had painstakingly styled her hair and applied cosmetics with the skill and precision of a professional stylist. The striking colour choices and absolute meticulousness would suggest this was someone who wanted to be noticed, wanted to attract people's attention. A photo of Belle's head and shoulders, if posted on social media, would be the kind of image that would invite hundreds of 'likes'. I wondered if she used social media and thought that probably she didn't. I'd heard she was reclusive, and her presentation struck me as shut off. However, Belle's choice of clothes, while equally well-thought through and co-ordinated, suggested someone who wanted *not* to be seen and *not* to attract attention.

I had a sense of Belle's clothes as armour, or what Esther Bick called a 'second skin' (Bick, 1968). Bick was a Polish-born, London-trained psychoanalyst, who was analysed herself by Michael Balint and later by Melanie Klein. She became head of the child psychotherapy training at the Tavistock Clinic, and her work has been of great significance to child psychotherapy trainees. Bick introduced the concept of infant observation to clinical trainings, which involves the student therapist observing a baby from soon after birth for the first two years of its life, once a week, for one hour. To those who haven't undertaken an infant observation, the notion of silently watching a baby, without interacting in any way, for an hour a week may sound bizarre and painstaking. For those of us who have done it, it certainly starts out as bizarre and painstaking, but then it develops into the most worthwhile and enriching learning experience and equips therapists with the skills to really observe the minutiae of what's going on. I think that this capacity to observe the minutiae is one of the fundamental competences in the psychotherapists' armoury.

Something that Bick observed was the significance of containment. She thought of the baby's skin as its primary container – literally, the bag that holds the baby together. The containing presence of the mother is what allows the baby to develop what Bick called a 'psychic skin' – that is, a sense of itself as separate, safe and held in the mind of another. If this early experience of maternal containment isn't experienced as good enough, the baby has a sense of being *un*contained and in danger of falling apart. Such experiences are what lead to the development of a 'second skin', which is a psychological defence against the fear of not being contained and a primitive attempt at self-containment.

According to psychoanalytic theory, this second skin defence is a psychological construct established to defend against disintegration or falling apart and symbolises a type of 'pseudo' independence (Mellier, 2014). Pseudo because, while the infant might look like they are independent and self-sufficient, they are merely responding to the sense they have that the person they need to depend upon is unavailable.

The concept of a second skin defence came to mind when I met Belle. I had a sense of her holding herself together with protective layers of clothing, and it was also my sense from observing her presentation. She sat stock still, perched on the edge of her seat, feet planted firmly in the floor and hands planted firmly on her knees. She stared straight ahead in my direction, but I felt she was looking but not really seeing me, and her gaze remained mostly fixed and mostly unchanged. I think that this too symbolised an effort to hold herself together. Consider the act of balancing on one leg: it's much easier if you set your eyes on a fixed point, which acts as an anchor and prevents you from falling over. If you allow your eyes to wander, you're more likely to wobble and fall. Belle seemed to need external anchors – heavy clothes, a motionless posture, a fixed stare – which made me wonder about her internal anchor – that is, her internal capacity to stay upright; to not wobble or fall over or fall apart.

Belle didn't say much in that first meeting. I hadn't expected her to, if I'm honest. It was mostly a factual discussion between her mother and me about her developmental history, in her presence. I'd heard some of the more recent story from Emmy while Belle was still in hospital, but during the consultation I asked about the pregnancy and birth, and about Belle's childhood and developmental milestones. There seemed to be nothing unusual. The pregnancy and birth were described as 'normal' and Belle's early years were said to be 'ordinary', according to her mother. If anything, Belle achieved her milestones earlier than anticipated and seemed 'advanced for her age'. I wondered if this was actually the case or a further illustration of pseudo independence. I noticed that Emmy was respectful of her daughter and checked in with her regularly, with 'The way I remember it is…' and '…I hope it's okay to say…' kinds of statements.

When Belle did speak, she did so in a barely audible voice that sounded as if it belonged to a little girl, rather than a 16-year-old young woman. Emmy's description of 'just a little girl' floated into my awareness and I asked myself how old she seemed to me now; could it be 12? From the story presented, it certainly seemed that Belle had had a flying start in life, 'until something happened suddenly…' (Laufer & Laufer, 1995) and then she'd got stuck. I was curious about what had precipitated the stuck-ness.

The power of projection

I'd already learned, from consulting with Emmy, that 12 was a significant number in the family narrative. It was Belle's age when her mother first became consciously aware of her daughter's suicidal behaviour; it was the age Emmy had been when her father left; it was the number of weeks pregnant Emmy was when she lost her first pregnancy, and also, I now realised, it was the number of years later that she had become pregnant with Belle. I wondered what that experience might have been like for Emmy – her second pregnancy, masquerading as her first. I fantasised that the earlier traumatic experience of loss could have been re-enacted in her pregnancy with Belle; that the fear of the same thing happening again, this time to a planned and hoped-for pregnancy, might have somehow *got into* her baby.

In psychoanalytic terms, frightened and frightening feelings are projected rather than contained (J. Williams, 1997). I wondered if this concept could go some way towards making sense of Belle's lack of an internal capacity to hold herself together, and of her suicidal behaviour. Perhaps her apparent pseudo independence had developed in response to a sense of a mother who projected rather than contained anxious and frightening feelings. This projected fear of loss, re-enacted in suicidal behaviour, had become recognisable to Emmy only when Belle reached 12 years old. I wondered if this awareness symbolised an unconscious act of repetition – the tendency to repeat both pleasurable and painful experiences (Freud, 1920). Had Emmy become so alert to and so frightened about her second 'baby' dying at 12 years because of the experience she'd endured of her first 'baby' dying at 12 weeks? Possibly. The seemingly unconnected knowledge I had learned from Emmy and observed in Belle was starting to join up and make some sense.

Psychodynamic psychotherapists in particular are alert to the idea that the presentation of the child (at any age) often expresses the parent's unconscious conflict (Brazelton & Cramer, 1990). It's crucial to point out here, as I have elsewhere, that this isn't about blaming; it's about making sense of. It is not unusual, in my clinical experience, to come across a young person whose presentation doesn't seem to 'fit', and it can sometimes feel as if they are presenting on behalf of somebody else. I might get a sense with an anxious young person, for example, that it's not *their* anxiety I'm witnessing, or with a young person presenting ritualised behaviours that it's not *their* compulsion that's being played out. These types of presentation symbolise a repetition of the parent's traumatic past in the present: what psychoanalysts might refer to as 'ghosts in the nursery' (Fraiberg et al., 1975).

I had a hypothesis that Belle's depression and suicidal presentation were the ghosts in the nursery that contained fragments of her mother's history, but what use was my hypothesis and my psychoanalytic learning to them? In theoretical terms, probably not much use at all; but in terms of offering Belle a sense that she was being thought about and understood, it could be very useful indeed. An often-repeated refrain of adolescence goes something along the lines of 'My parents just don't get it'. I can get it for young people and let them know that I get it and eventually witness them feeling that I get it, and these are some of the most valuable things that happen in my therapy room. That feeling a young person gets when they feel understood is magical. As with lots of feelings, it's hard to put that felt sense into words, but I recognise it when it happens and, most importantly, so do they.

Wanting to die

Belle arrived in therapy highly defended by her second skin armour, fixed gaze and rigid thoughts. Those defences were the things that were holding her together and so it was important to respect them and let them be; to observe them and acknowledge them and not attempt to dismantle them. It was those defences that were keeping Belle alive. I think the potential of death, somewhat paradoxically, was keeping Belle alive too. I understood this in terms of a kind of escape lane, like those on steep hills, where vehicles can stop in a pile of sand if their brakes fail. So long as Belle had a potential way out – death – she could keep on living. That's not to say I didn't take her suicidal ideation seriously. The reality of danger to life, just like the risk of a vehicle's brakes failing on a steep hill, is a constant threat because of its 'internally determined compelling quality' (Laufer & Laufer, 1995, p.120).

Anyone who's worked with a depressed and suicidal young person will know how painful the process is. Most sessions, Belle sat fixed and rigid, responding in barely audible monosyllables or barely visible blinks of the eye. Any efforts I made to engage her verbally were met with phrases such as, 'I don't know' or, 'I'm not sure' or, 'I feel the same'. At first, I found it difficult to sit with the emptiness of the sessions, unbearable even, and felt compelled to fill the silence, to try to pull her out of it and out of her depression. This isn't like me; I'm usually comfortable enough with silence. When I reflected on what might be going on, I realised that I was being pulled into behaving like Emmy, the mother who so desperately wanted her daughter to be 'a normal little girl' again, engaged rather than withdrawn, and alive rather than dead. Once I'd noticed this, I was able to be more like me: to be in the unbearable silence with Belle and to feel what that felt like. It felt awful. It felt frightening. Sometimes, it felt overwhelming. Most weeks, when I closed the door as Belle left her session, I was filled up with unbearable dread that I wouldn't see her again because she would be dead. I think this illustrated the reality of Belle's potential to repeat the suicidal act, but also, perhaps, something of Emmy's unbearable dread that she could lose her 'baby'.

My therapeutic role, in those slow, empty, painful weeks that turned into months, was to provide a holding function – to hold what was going on for me and for Belle and to hold the unbearableness of it all, so that Belle (and Emmy) didn't have to hold it all by themselves. I also held onto the hope, which wasn't always easy and sometimes ebbed and flowed, but I think that's an important part of my role as a psychotherapist too. When situations feel desperate and unbearable and totally hope*less* for young people and their families, I can hold onto the hope until a time when they are able to do so. I believe that there is always hope in anyone who engages in therapy, even if it's the tiniest spark, because why else would they come? Spring flowers bloom again after the darkest, coldest winters when it sometimes feels impossible to believe that they will. Their roots and shoots are dormant for months but, given the right amounts of light and warmth and nutrients, they flourish. I sometimes thought of Belle as a dormant spring flower, and I never stopped believing that she would emerge from her winter slumber.

Daring to live

The first signs of emergent growth came many months after I'd first met Belle. There were minuscule, almost imperceptible shifts that my experience of infant observation had trained me to notice. I remember watching that infant, during my training, as he started learning to walk. First, he used both hands to hold onto the furniture, levering himself up with the strength of his arms, delighted to be off the floor, propelled to a new, elevated position all by himself. Then he learned he could move himself, still in an upright position, by holding on with his hands and shuffling his hips and legs, toppling over when he ran out of something to hold onto, then pulling himself up and trying again. Over time, and with increased confidence, the infant could be encouraged to relinquish his grip on the furniture and take his first steps unaided, into the open, containing arms of his parent.

This experimentation with holding on and letting go is what came to mind in my session with Belle, about 10 months into therapy. I had a feeling that she had let go of me with her eyes. It was subtle, but I noticed it. And it happened again the week after and the week after that, when she also moved her hands off her lap and sat further back in the chair. It was as if Belle had been able to relinquish the rigid holding on, because she had internalised a sense of being held (G. Williams, 1997). The shifts were subtle, but I was as ecstatic as a parent whose child has just learnt to stand on their own two feet. I was also cautious, knowing that 'a new peacefulness, or a sense of relief that things appear to be resolved… may, paradoxically, be a cause for increased concern' (Parker & Eyers, 2010, p.30). I decided to share with Belle what I had observed about her.

'I've noticed something different these last few sessions…'
'Have you?'

'Yes, it's felt different. You've seemed different.'

'Have I?'

'I think so. I wonder if you've felt different?'

'Maybe. A little.'

'Yes, the differences I've noticed and felt have been little too.' I wanted Belle to know we'd experienced the same 'little' shifts. I didn't want to alarm her with anything too 'big'.

'I wonder if you can put into words those little differences that you feel, Belle?'

'I'm not sure...'

'Okay. Would you like me to go first?'

'Yes, please.'

I didn't want Belle to feel pressured, but I also didn't want this moment to pass us by unacknowledged. We'd worked at her pace, danced to her tune, for almost a year. The dance had been slow, excruciatingly slow at times, and I needed to be certain that she was ready for a change in tempo. So, I told her what I'd observed about her when we'd first met: her very still posture, her fixed stare, her little voice, and how I'd noticed a shift in the way she sat, the way she looked at me and around the room, and how she spoke. I observed Belle carefully as I spoke, gauging whether she felt comfortable enough to hear more, like a mother deciding when her infant has had enough play or stimuli or walking practice. Just as mothers (usually) learn the rhythms of their babies by watching, responding and prolonging their attention, looking for cues and matching their responses accordingly (Brazelton & Cramer, 1990), so too do psychotherapists (usually) learn the rhythms of our clients by observing, responding and attending to them. We think and we feel, process and contain, and finally, when it feels right to do so, we give back our digested, processed thoughts in a digestible, processable form. Belle's response told me she was ready.

'I've noticed that too. I've noticed that I feel more comfortable now. More relaxed. I feel calmer.'

'Can you say more about that, Belle, to help me understand how you feel?'

'I still think about suicide but it's not always my first thought when I wake up in the morning or my last thought before I go to sleep at night. I used to think, okay, I've not done it today, I can do it tomorrow. I used to think that every day. And in the morning, I'd think, I'll not do it straight away, but maybe later. And that's how I would get through the days. There are some days now that I realise, I haven't thought about killing myself at all until I'm ready to go to sleep, and then I think, okay, well, I didn't think about it today, there's no point in thinking about it now, and maybe I won't think about it tomorrow either.'

I'd never heard Belle say so many words. To continue the symbolism of the infant taking its first wobbly steps, it was as if Belle had just walked the entire length of the garden! She said more, in quantity as well as quality, in that response than she had in the 10 months preceding it. I think she could tell from my facial expression that I was amazed and mesmerised and excited. And I think she was a little bit amazed too: that she'd thought all those thoughts and that she'd shared them with me and what that might mean. I ventured a theory.

'It sounds to me, Belle, as if there is a bigger part of you, or at least a slightly less little part of you than before, that doesn't want to die.'

'Yes, I think there is.'

'A part of you that wants to live, perhaps?' I tentatively enquired.

'Yes.'

'And is hopeful that you will?'

'Yes.'

'That's so pleasing to know. For both of us, I think.'

'Yes, it is.'

Just being

Throughout many painful, frightening, unbearable months, Belle and I spent dozens of excruciatingly slow, therapeutic hours together, with neither of us saying or apparently doing very much, apart from just being there with each other. Or at least that's how it might have looked to an untrained eye. What I'd actually been doing was feeling my feelings about Belle and thinking my thoughts with her, and processing those thoughts and feelings in order to give Belle the opportunity of having 'an emotional experience rather than an intellectual one' (Gray, 2014, p.43). This enabled her to feel her feelings and think her thoughts too, in the presence of an attentive 'other'. I also believe that Belle had had a simultaneous experience at home, giving her the sense of being held by an attentive 'mother'.

I hadn't been Emmy's psychotherapist, but I'd applied my psychotherapeutic thinking to make sense of her story in relation to Belle, and I'd used psychotherapeutic skills to acknowledge her experiences and validate her feeling responses. Together, we had explored Emmy's past in order to set the context for Belle's present. We had made sense of the mother–daughter relationship in reality as well as in unconscious fantasy, by illuminating themes, patterns, family scripts and 'ghosts in the nursery'. And, in doing so, we had freed up Emmy to accept a new narrative in which she wasn't blindly or unconsciously compelled to repeat the past.

I had fantasised that Belle's depression and repeated suicidal behaviour might not have belonged to her, but might have, in some unconscious way, *got into her*, through her mother's projections of frightened and frightening feelings. Through her admirable honesty and capacity for reflection, Emmy had been able to think about this with me too, and had made sense of it and become less controlled by it, freeing her up to offer a more containing function to her daughter. In turn, Belle had been freed of her second-skin defences and pseudo independence. She had been able to relinquish the rigid holding on because she had internalised a sense of being held by her mother and by me. She no longer felt defeated or trapped, hopeless or desperate. She didn't need the escape lane of suicide. She wasn't acting out her mother's projections. She was ready to live.

9

Bored and angry (but mostly angry)

Connie, Saskia, Chantelle, Mo and Mercedes are bored and angry. There are concerns about their lack of engagement in school and their risk-taking behaviour out of school. Can group work help them make sense of how they feel, improve their sense of self-worth and open the door to change?

. . . .

'I'm bored.'
'Same.'
'This so fucking boring.'
'I know.'
'Life is so fucking boring.'
'You're so right.'
'There's literally *nothing* to do.'
'And literally *nothing* to look forward to.'
'What's the point?'
'There is no point.'
'Literally.'
'I know, right.'
'Life is like, So. Fucking. B-O-R-I-N-G.'

This was the opening gambit in my first session with this new group of 16-year-old girls. Connie was bored. Saskia was bored too. Chantelle agreed that life was boring, and so did Mo, who literally spelled it out for us. Mercedes, who you might remember from the Introduction, was seemingly too bored to say anything, for now. These bored Year-11 girls had been referred to me because their student support manager was worried about their lack of engagement in school and their risk-taking behaviour out of school. In a candid conversation, she told me she was concerned they would 'fuck up, drop out, and fuck up some more'. They were deemed to be 'at risk' – of failing, dropping out and getting into serious trouble of the drugs, alcohol or teenage pregnancy kind. Our group sessions ran for the duration of one school term. The girls were typically challenging and regularly boisterous. Progress was by no means linear or sequential; sometimes it was hard for me to recognise any progress at all. What I'm sharing in this chapter is a tidied up, thought-through version of events, rather than a chronological one. I am hoping it presents a flavour of the chaos, with the benefit of reflective hindsight.

'You're bored,' I said, stating the obvious.

'We're *so* fucking bored,' Saskia agreed.

'In general, or about something in particular?' I asked.

'In general,' Saskia clarified. 'Everything is so boring.'

'Everything?'

'Yeah, everything.' She seemed adamant.

'Okay… I wonder what would make everything seem a bit less boring?'

'Nothing would. It's just all so fucking boring.'

'Okay, I get it,' I said.

'No, you don't!' Chantelle challenged me.

'Don't I?'

'No!'

'How come?'

'How can you?' she asked.

'How can I?'

'What are you, a fucking parrot or something?'

'I'm not a parrot, no,' I stated, as calmly as I could. 'I'm just trying to understand what you mean. Maybe you can help me?'

'I thought you were meant to help us!'

'Did you?'

'Isn't that why we're all here, in this fucking boring fucking group, so you can help us to *not* be so fucking bored?'

'Is that why you think we're here, for me to help you not be so bored?'

Chantelle shrugged.

'What does everyone else think?'

Silence descended.

'What about you, Connie. Can you say why you think we're here?'

She shrugged too.

'What about you, Saskia?'
No response.
'Mercedes?'
She proffered a grunt.
'Mo, any offers?'
'I haven't got a fucking clue,' she said in a sing-song sort of voice.
At least Mo was talking to me, and as it was the most promising connection I had at that moment, I decided to pursue it.
'I'm interested in that, Mo, that you came here even though you haven't got a fucking clue why you came.'
She side-eyed me suspiciously, probably because I'd said 'fucking', but she didn't say anything else.
'I'm wondering if that's the same for everyone else.'
'What?' Saskia asked, as if she'd just woken up.
'I said I noticed that you all came here, but I was wondering if, like Mo, you don't know why?'
'Suppose so,' Saskia admitted.
'That's interesting,' I repeated.
'God, your life must be as fucking boring as ours if you find *this* shit interesting!'
I smiled. 'I do find it interesting. I'm really interested in getting to know why each of you came to the group.'
'And you're interested in that because…?' Mo goaded.
'Good question, Mo. Why am I interested…?' I was playing for time as I thought aloud and she knew it. 'Well, I suppose I'm curious why you would do something without having a good reason to do it.'
'Fuck knows!' Mo spluttered.
'But do *you* know, Mo? Do *you* know why you came?'
Chantelle tried to help her out. 'It's not like we had a choice, is it?'
'Isn't it?'
'No, she's right. We got sent here.'
'Who sent you?'
'That woman in pastoral… what's her name?'
'Miss Martinez?'
'Yeah, her.'
Everyone nodded.
'I know I've only known you all for, what…' I glanced at the clock, '10 minutes…' – is that all it was? It felt like longer – 'but you don't strike me as girls who would do anything you didn't want to, even if

you were "sent" by a teacher.' I put air quotes around 'sent' to make my point.

They all stared blankly, either at me or at the floor, and so I continued.

'So, if that's true, that you're not those sorts of girls, it makes me think there must be a part of each of you that thought it might be worthwhile to come.'

'I wouldn't have bothered if I'd know it would be like this,' Mo stated.

'Like what?' I wondered.

'Fucking boring', she clarified, like it should be obvious.

'Same,' Saskia and Connie agreed, simultaneously. Chantelle and Mercedes said nothing.

'Ah yes, the issue of boring. Tell me about that. Tell me what boring means to you?' I encouraged them.

'Boring means fucking boring! Jeez, are you dumb or something? What's the fucking point?' Saskia spat out the words and then sank down further on her chair to the point where it looked as if she might slide off.

What *was* the point? I was beginning to ask myself the same question.

'Well, I wonder if we could unpick that a bit.'

'Ooh, yes, let's unpick it,' Saskia mocked, miming pinching movements in the air with her fingers. A couple of the girls sniggered, a couple snarled; I don't remember who did what. I decided to be less wondering and more directive. I persevered.

'Maybe we could each say something about the different parts of our life: school, social stuff, family perhaps, and share the most boring thing and the least boring thing. Could we give that a try?'

I was relieved when Mo took the initiative. 'That's easy,' she began. 'Everything about school is boring. Everything about home is boring. And everything about my social life is boring.'

Chantelle followed suit: 'School and home are totally boring.'

'And your social life?' I asked.

'What fucking social life?'

'You don't have a social life?'

'No.'

Mercedes had so far been silent. I'd similarly experienced her as non-verbal the first time I'd met her, in the one individual meeting we'd had, when she'd been sent to me for 'anger management'. But she'd accepted my invitation to join the group, and so I tried again to engage her.

'How would you describe school, Mercedes?'

'Fuck off.' Her response was abrupt, but it was familiar.

'And home?'

'Fuck off.'

'Your social life?'

'Will. You. Just. Fuck. Off.'

I commented that Mercedes didn't seem up for talking much today and she told me, 'No fucking shit, Sherlock,' which elicited a ripple of sniggers from the other girls. She was replaying the lines she'd spat out at me the first time we'd met, but this time with an audience.

I took a moment to reflect on what her responses had provoked in me and, if I'm honest, it was an eagerness to find out more. She had spirit. She had fire in her belly. She was rebellious, unpredictable and not afraid to say what she thought. I could imagine what she might achieve if she channelled those traits into something worthwhile, rather than challenging me and/or playing to the crowd. I was really keen to work with them all, to bring them on board, engage them, get to know them, make sense of them and, ultimately, help them. I wasn't going to just fuck off, I was going to stick with them.

Let's be honest

I decided to share my feeling response with the group. 'At the risk of stating the obvious, *again*...' I glanced at Mercedes, who was glaring at the floor. 'I'm sensing that so far I might have missed the mark a bit here.'

A couple of girls shuffled in their chairs; the others remained stock still.

'I'm grateful that you've each been honest with me about how you're feeling, which seems to mostly be bored, but also, I think, a bit pissed off... with home, school, maybe Miss Martinez, maybe me. One thing that's really important is that we feel safe enough to be honest with each other here, so I'm pleased you were able to do that.'

They were still listening, and no one had told me to fuck off, so I continued.

'My understanding about why Miss Martinez suggested the group to the five of you in particular is because she's noticed that you seem bored too and she's worried about you and about your behaviour.' I noticed Saskia and Chantelle squirm. 'I'm not here to judge you. I'm hoping that you will start to feel a bit better about life, a bit less bored and a bit less angry perhaps.' I still had their attention. 'I'm going to be honest with you too. I'm really keen to get to know you all, to learn more about you, what you enjoy, what you don't enjoy, maybe what you're finding tough, what's *really* pissing you off.'

'*You're* starting to piss me off!' Saskia stopped me in my tracks.

'Am I?' I had thought I was doing okay. 'How am I pissing you off?'

'By going on and on and fucking on…'

'I suppose it might seem like that. It's just that it felt important to say those things and to be honest with you all.'

'Yeah, thanks, Miss,' Connie said, 'I do actually appreciate that.'

'That's okay, Connie. And you can call me Jeanine. You can *all* call me Jeanine.'

Saskia accused Connie of being a 'suck up', Connie gave as good as she got. Chantelle sided with Saskia and Mo argued for Connie. Mercedes observed in silence. She seemed to do that a lot. I noticed her observing me too, which I'd experienced before, of course, when she'd perceived my barely-there smile and gentle nod of the head, and delivered the immortal line, 'Will you stop fucking nodding!' I let things play out for a while, ready to step in if it got out of hand, and then I commented on what I'd observed.

'It's interesting to watch what happens when you have a disagreement.'

'Is it?'

'Yes.'

'Okay. That's weird,' Chantelle squirmed.

'I'm going to stick with interesting rather than weird.' I took a risk and asked Mercedes if she'd found it interesting too.

'It was fascinating!'

That was a better reaction than I'd anticipated, although I was worried there was a chance she was being sarcastic. 'Go on…' I encouraged her, 'What did you find fascinating?'

'How they all have positions.' I nodded for her to continue.

'Saskia's clearly the gobby one.'

'Oh, thanks,' Saskia said, mock offended.

'Sorry, but you are.'

'I know, fair point,' she conceded.

'As I was saying,' Mercedes paused for comic effect, 'Saskia's the gobby one, but Mo likes to be in charge, so they clash. Chantelle is a follower, and *she's* the real suck up, to whoever she thinks has the power. And I'm not sure about Connie; she's a bit of a dark horse.'

'I don't think you're allowed to say "dark horse" any more,' Connie challenged. 'It's racist.'

'How can it be fucking racist, Connie, when I'm black and you're white?'

'Oh, okay. Good point.' Connie backed down.

I invited the others to share their response to the way Mercedes had described them. Saskia agreed that she was gobby and Mo said she liked to be in charge. Chantelle gave a 'I can't argue with that' kind of expression when she was described as a follower, and Connie wasn't sure what it was like not to have a 'position'. I think she felt a bit put out. Mercedes seemed spot on and, because she was their peer, the girls had taken her straight-talking, honest observations at face value. I really wanted to know how it felt to be noticed in this way, but I didn't think the girls were ready to acknowledge their feelings just yet; I didn't think they had the words, other than 'bored' or 'angry' or 'I don't know' – another adolescent stock answer. But often 16-year-olds *don't* know how they feel, or why they did what they did, or what they want to do in the future, and while that's often frustrating for adults, it's even more agonising for adolescents, who hate not knowing (Luxmoore, 2010).

'Thank you for sharing your observations, Mercedes. And thank you, girls, for listening. I think this is the sort of thing that might turn out to be helpful.'

'Arguing?' Chantelle asked.

'Noticing, being noticed, talking, listening...'

'And that will help us *how*, exactly?' Mo pressed.

'Well, hopefully by noticing yourselves and each other, and how you relate to each other here, you will get a better understanding of what's going on for you – a better sense of why you feel the way you feel and why you're doing the stuff you're doing.'

'What about you?' she asked.

'Me?'

'Yes, you. Will *you* be telling us why *you* feel the way you do and why *you're* doing what you're doing?'

'I like that question, Mo.'

'Teachers always say that when they aren't going to answer you, "*That's a really good question but...*",' she mimicked.

'First, I'm not a teacher, so teacher rules don't apply to me.' I admit, I delivered that remark with a small sense of victory. 'Second, I'm very happy to answer your question. I will absolutely be sharing with you how I feel in response to what I notice happening in the group. But I won't be telling you about what I do outside of the group because this space is about you, not me.'

'How is *that* fucking fair?' Saskia demanded.

'I think it's absolutely fair that I don't bring my stuff here. This is *your* space. I'm here to help you, not the other way around, as Chantelle reminded us earlier. If I started talking about my stuff, then it would become about me, and that would be really unfair on all of you.'

'Sounds like a cop-out if you ask me,' Mo stated. 'You expect us to tell you everything and you tell us fuck-all in return.'

'I really don't expect you to tell me everything, Mo, only what you're comfortable with. Like I said, it would be totally unfair of me to talk about myself here, when I'm sure you all have enough on your plates. This is a space where you don't have to worry about me or how what you do or say affects me.'

'Because you don't give a shit?' Saskia half stated/half asked.

'I absolutely do give a shit. I give a very large shit about every one of you. Okay, that sounded weird. What I mean is, I'm not your teacher, or your parent, or your friend, so you don't need to worry about how what you say affects me. It won't change me, or our relationship or how I feel about you.'

'Now she's gone all lovey-do-da on us!' Connie said, and the others laughed, but not in a ridiculing way – in a more affirmative, non-threatening way. I thought it seemed as if they liked the idea of being liked, maybe even loved the notion of being loved. It might not be too much of a stretch to imagine that they could love the idea of being loved by me.

Falling in love

Adolescents talk about love all the time. As veteran child counsellor and writer Nick Luxmoore said, 'They're searching for it, basking in it, never finding it, losing it, not trusting it, being transformed by it...' (Luxmoore, 2019). But love can be elusive, because, as any parent or professional will tell you, adolescents can be hard to love. By now, it should be blatantly obvious which side of the mast my colours are nailed to, but I can see their point. Once puberty hits (or just prior), many teens (or 'tweens') become selfish, self-indulgent, self-obsessed, self-centred, self-seeking, self-serving, omnipotent narcissists, which doesn't make them very easy to love. That might sound harsh but it's true and, furthermore, adolescents can't help it. In part, this bolstered-up sense of self-importance communicates something of their fragility; their omnipotent 'bigness' is a defence against feeling small and vulnerable (Waddell, 2018); their 'gang mentality' is a defence against loneliness; their seemingly selfish narcissism is an attempt to restore a fragile sense of self. In other words, as I've repeated hundreds of times before, the physical and verbal behaviour we witness on the outside is a manifestation of the thoughts and feelings on the inside, and for many adolescents, the strongest communication of all is 'I want to be loveable'.

On the face of it, this might seem to be in conflict with the central task of adolescence, which is separation – a paradox demonstrated by the push/pull type of relating that I frequently hear about in therapy. A young person tells me in session that they've met someone; they're *amazing*, but they're taking it slowly. Then, they can't help themselves, they're all in, they think they're in love, this person is fucking amazing! Actually, they're not so great, now they think about it; they're a bit of a dick, actually, and they fucking hate them; how could they have been so stupid? I experience it first-hand too, in the here and now of the therapeutic relationship: one minute they're invested, I'm the best thing since sliced bread, they're telling me that they're telling me more than they've ever told anyone, ever before. The next minute, they want to leave, what time to do we finish, and why am I making them come here and they're not telling me anything else and I'm a shit therapist and they fucking hate this and 'Will you stop fucking nodding'.

Sometimes, as with this group, young people start from a position of hating it/me and move towards a place where they invest in the relationship, but usually adolescents flip-flop between the two positions of loving and hating. It was the child psychoanalyst Melanie Klein who identified the fundamental principle of ambivalence in psychoanalytic theory. She suggested that the baby both loves its mother (when she provides what s/he needs) and hates her (when she doesn't), and asserted that the mother absorbs the baby's feelings and, in turn, both loves and hates the baby too (Klein, 1957). The same is true of adolescents, who love their parents/teachers/therapists when they are perceived as giving, and hate them when they're perceived as withholding.

These feelings are natural. They are natural for parents/teachers/therapists too, but if there's one thing that seems to be misunderstood and derided more than loving the young people we support, it's hating them. Parents, and those *in loco parentis,* are expected to be automatons, programmed only to feel benevolent feelings and 'unconditional positive regard' (Rogers, 1961). 'Bad' people feel hate. 'Good' people feel love. This is the stuff of fairy tales, not real life. In real life, we (whoever we are) meet people we like, people who push our buttons, people we love and people we hate. Some of those people are young. Some of them are our own children. Some of them are our clients. It's important to acknowledge the gamut of feelings we feel, own them, and work through them in private reflection, personal therapy and/or supervision, just as we invite young people to do in therapy. It's important that we practise what we preach.

The push/pull, love/hate, ambivalent style of relating I experience in relationship with adolescents makes sense. They want to be loved, but they can't just come right out and say it, because that would make them vulnerable, and they already feel vulnerable and fragmented, and relationships are fragile, and they already feel fragile, and they want to feel strong and whole and special and loved and fucking hell, adolescence is so excruciating. It's even more excruciating for young people whose early experiences have been less than good enough, those who've already experienced rejection, abandonment, trauma, neglect or abuse. How can we expect them to make and maintain a relationship, or feel loved and loveable, when they know how badly that can turn out? How can they expect that of themselves? How can they take that kind of risk? Those young people – the Mercedes, Mos, Saskias, Connies and Chantelles of the world – act like they hate everyone, trust no one and expect everyone to leave. That's why they're so angry. That's why they present as adversarial and antagonistic. Their behaviour is intended to challenge us, because they are throwing down the gauntlet to see what we will do. Will we argue and fight back, stay and work it out, or just fuck off? But even as they're telling us to fuck off, they are hoping that we'll stay and work it out.

Our first experience of being in a relationship happens in infancy. If it is good enough, social and emotional intelligence follows. If that first relationship is chaotic, if life is a mess, children develop messy feelings and recreate a messy life by (re-)creating havoc. They are less able to differentiate or fine tune their feelings (so they only recognise extreme or all-purpose feelings like 'bored' or 'angry'); they are socially awkward, confused and incompetent, which manifests in aggression or withdrawal or both (Jennings, 2011). We cannot undo the past, of course; we cannot turn back the clock and give adolescents a less chaotic, more loving start in life, with a more finely attuned maternal attachment, and we cannot become the parents our clients may have wanted (Gray, 2014). We have to accept the reality (and help them to accept it too) – that they live in an imperfect world, full of disappointments and boredom and things that will make them angry. But we can give them the opportunity to experience a different kind of relationship with a different kind of 'parental figure' – a relationship that is healthy, respectful and loving with someone who values their needs and wishes above their own. In other words, we can show them unconditional love, no matter what they throw at us.

Some people have challenged my use of 'love' to describe my feelings towards adolescent clients. In contrast, others have asked, 'How can you do what you do without getting attached to the young people you work with?' My answer is, 'I can't, and if I didn't get attached to them, I don't think I would be doing a very good job.' Love is about affection and attachment, and the therapeutic relationship (like the adolescent) needs both of these elements to thrive. The Oxford English Dictionary defines love as 'A feeling or disposition of deep affection or fondness for someone… manifesting itself in concern for the other's welfare and pleasure in his or her presence (distinguished from sexual love); great liking, strong emotional attachment; a feeling or disposition of benevolent attachment' (Oxford English Dictionary, 2021). This absolutely sums up my sense of the therapeutic relationships I have with adolescents. I hope it goes without saying that what I feel for them is different to the love I feel for a romantic partner, family member or friend, but there is no denying that it is a kind of love, both contained by therapeutic boundaries and providing the container itself.

Winnicott reminds us that physical holding is the way that a mother demonstrates her love for her baby (Winnicott, 1965b), which is akin, I believe, to the kind of loving, therapeutic holding we can offer to young people. Just as there are mothers who do and do not have the ability to hold their babies, there are therapists who do and do not have the capacity to lovingly hold adolescents (Luxmoore, 2019), which may have something to do with their own experiences of being held (or not) as babies and/or their own experiences of being held lovingly (or not) as clients in their own personal therapy. Love has a long history in psychoanalytic literature. Coltart believed that it was the informing energy at the heart of therapy (Coltart, 1993). Ferenczi asserted that 'it is the physician's love that heals the patient' (Suttie, 1935, p.75), and Freud is quoted as saying (as early as 1906) that 'psychoanalysis is a cure through love' (Freud Museum, 2018). I concur. I don't embrace young people physically, but I hold them emotionally and symbolically, with enough love to enable them to feel safe and contained. Love without technique is potentially dangerous and un-containing (Luxmoore, 2019), but therapy without love is a soulless, mechanical, technique-driven, box-ticking encounter – and adolescents will sense that a mile off.

What's the point?

It is important that any therapeutic relationship feels safe, and this should not be taken for granted. Moreover, the relationship should be given time to develop, particularly if young people are not used to feeling held and loved. Boundaries are a fundamentally important part of any therapeutic relationship, whether that's one-to-one, family or group work, and they enable the development of that sense of safety. In a group, there are the traditional boundaries of frequency, duration and setting that we might think of as the 'therapeutic frame' (Gray, 1994), as well as boundaries around personal space. There is also the boundary of confidentiality, and an agreement that what is said in the group stays in the group, with the usual exceptions of supervision and safeguarding. Another 'technical' concern relates to the purpose of the group: the 'Why are we meeting?' question, or, as Mo or Mercedes might have put it, 'What's the point?' When a group meets, it does so for a specific task and has an impulse to work and collaborate (Bion, 1961). Connie, Saskia, Chantelle, Mo and Mercedes were initially uncertain about the group task, but that didn't matter; they showed up and they joined in, and in a way, 'becoming a group [was] the therapy' (Reid, 1999). That was the task in and of itself.

From a theoretical perspective, the primary task could be defined as providing a container where the group of 16-year-olds could explore their thoughts and feelings, about self and others, while enduring whatever difficulties might arise within and between them. The young women exhibited behaviours, feelings, thoughts, words and emotions that at first appeared to spill out in a messy way: they argued, they complained, they challenged and they attacked – sometimes each other, but mostly me. These attacks could be perceived as an impulse against the primary task, conscious or unconscious, based on the desire to protect themselves from the anxiety associated with being in relationship (Roberts, 1994). I think that's partly true, but I also think the girls presented in a messy and chaotic way because it was all that they knew. Their life experiences had been messy and chaotic, and they were predisposed to repeat those experiences.

Young people express messy and chaotic experiences in a variety of ways: through embodiment (such as attacks on the self or others), taking on the role of destroyer (bully) or destroyed (bullied), or through projection (Jennings, 1998). I had been informed of these types of manifestations in each of the girl's lives. But the group experience was different to their real-life experiences in that what 'spilled out' could be noticed, thought about and worked through, rather than met with judgement, punishment, retaliation or rejection. And if what was mirrored back to them was different (and more loving), clinical experience had taught me that what 'spilled out' would become different too.

In therapeutic work (both individual and in groups), young people have an experience of feeling held, when the therapist is able to 'hold' them in their mind. For an adolescent who was denied the experience of being held in their mother's mind as an infant, this can be an unfamiliar experience. Unfamiliar can feel threatening. Threatening can provoke the need to defend themselves by using an attack, such as telling the therapist to fuck off, or stop fucking nodding. Over time – sometimes *lots* of time – the holding experience starts to feel less threatening and more containing, and the attacks recede. But it can still feel strange to be noticed or have your words or behaviours mirrored back to you 'like a fucking parrot', or have someone 'find your shit interesting', and to trust in the restorative process of being noticed and listened to.

Mo, Mercedes, Connie, Saskia and Chantelle shared their collective disbelief that participation in an experiential group, where all they were expected to do was turn up and be noticed, would bring about change. Mo had voiced this when she asked, 'And that will help us *how,* exactly?' In thinking about group processes, Bion states that a desire for an alternative to learning from experience is akin to a desire to arrive 'fully equipped as an adult' (Bion, 1961). I think this idea fits with the collective perception of adolescence. Adolescents want to skip to the part where they have all the liberties of adulthood and none of the restrictions of childhood without having to endure the transitionary period in between.

We're going on a bear hunt

Merely *being* 16 is a really tough ask for most 16-year-olds. Many of them struggle, in some way or other, and most have an understandable yearning to dodge the challenges and tribulations associated with this period of development. I think that getting through adolescence is a bit like going on Michael Rosen's infamous bear hunt (Rosen, 1993). Sixteen-year-olds might be offended that I'm referring to a book aimed at much younger children, for the reasons stated above – they want to be thought of as grown up – but I think the metaphors are fitting, and adolescence undeniably involves a certain amount of regression. It also involves plunging into 'deep cold rivers' of reality; the 'thick oozy mud' of sex and relationships; the 'big dark forests' of exams, pandemics and an uncertain future; the 'swirling whirling snowstorms' induced by natural hormones and artificial chemicals and the 'narrow gloomy caves' of loneliness and isolation. This is the ordinary, universal stuff of being 16, and, like the children on the bear hunt, all that young people can do is go through it. Psychotherapy can feel like going on a bear hunt too, and what we as therapists do is go through it with them.

So, if this is the ordinary experience of ordinary 16-year-olds (whatever ordinary means), what about those who have experienced adversity? Within the realm of child development studies, theorists make a distinction between 'circumstances that are sufficient to support normal child development' and those that 'chronically deprive the child of physical, emotional and intellectual stimulation or support, or pose an ongoing physical or emotional threat' (Asmussen et al., 2020), which require significant adaptation. What I am referring to here are adverse childhood experiences (ACEs). Ten ACEs have been identified by researchers as risk factors for physical, psychological, emotional and social difficulties in later life. These are: physical abuse, sexual abuse, verbal abuse, physical neglect, emotional neglect, a family member who is depressed or diagnosed with another mental illness, a family member who is addicted to alcohol or another substance, a family member who is in prison, witnessing a mother being abused, and losing a parent to separation, divorce or death. The latest research (in England) suggests that at least 2.5% of young people under 18 will experience some form of maltreatment or family dysfunction, while for those identified as children in need, the figure is 80%. Retrospective studies with adults suggest that 10–15% of the population have experienced four or more adverse experiences during their childhood (Asmussen et al., 2020), and four seems to be the 'magic number'.

Those adults who experienced four or more ACEs prior to their 18th birthday are twice as likely to develop obesity and diabetes; three times as likely to smoke, develop cancer, heart disease or respiratory disease; four times as likely to engage in sexual risk-taking and have mental health problems and problematic alcohol use, and seven times as likely to experience problematic drug use, interpersonal violence and self-harm (Asmussen et al., 2020). These statistics are startling, but they are also depressing, because we know this kind of data only represents what is known about and is likely to represent only the tip of the iceberg of what's really going on behind millions of closed doors in millions of homes.

Psychoeducation

As is the case for many of the young people referred to therapy, I suspected that Connie, Saskia, Chantelle, Mo and Mercedes might be experiencing some form of family dysfunction too. We'd been meeting for a few weeks when I decided to find out more, in an effort to contextualise the girls' presentations and help them to make sense of their boredom and anger. I began by asking a benign, open question.

'How was your weekend?'
Connie replied, 'The usual.'
'What's usual for you?'
'I got pissed.'
'And how was that?'
'A bit boring, to be honest.'
'Getting pissed is boring?'
'It is now. It's the same thing every weekend. We get a few bottles,

hang out, get pissed, something kicks off, we go home.'

'Did something kick off this weekend?'

'Yeah.'

'Can you tell us about that?' I enquired. 'Only if you want to,' I added, a bit wary about what she might divulge.

'One of the boys was getting a bit lairy. He can't handle his drink. He was grabbing at this girl who Declan's been talking to, so he knocked him out!'

'Your friend Declan knocked the lairy boy out?' I attempted to clarify.

'Yeah. Then the cops turned up and put him in a cell for the night. The other boy, I don't know his name, was taken away in an ambulance because he had concussion. We were all questioned about it. I told them what I saw, same as what I just told you.'

'I heard about that,' Chantelle said, her interest piqued, seemingly eager to know more.

'It sounds quite dramatic,' I suggested.

'Not really,' Connie disagreed.

'Not really?' I asked.

'Just the usual.'

'It's usual for someone to be arrested, someone else to be taken to hospital and for you to be questioned by the police?'

'Pretty much.'

'Is it usual for all of you?' I asked, attempting to open up the discussion.

'It's pretty standard, yeah,' Mo affirmed, nonplussed.

'We had the police at ours again on Sunday,' Saskia stated.

'For your dad?' Mo asked, as if she already knew the answer.

'Yeah.'

'Your dad was arrested on Sunday?' I checked.

'Yeah. He was off his fucking head. Smashed a window. I think the nosy bitch across the road called the cops. It's usually her.'

'Usually? Does this happen a lot?'

'Yeah. My dad's a complete wanker. He's always getting nicked.'

'Oh.' I didn't know what else to say.

'I thought he was inside,' Chantelle said, like it was the most ordinary thing in the world.

'He was. He's out now, but he'll go back in. It's like a revolving fucking door.'

Over the course of the session, I learned that Saskia's dad had served a number of short sentences for grievous bodily harm (GBH) and actual bodily harm (ABH), some of which had involved attacks on her mother. He was a heavy drinker and occasional drug user. Mercedes' brother was currently serving a sentence for aggravated burglary and possession of cannabis with intent to supply. The girls were familiar with the jargon. Like Saskia, Mercedes had also witnessed domestic abuse. Connie's mother used (illegal) cannabis for 'legit' medicinal reasons and had a diagnosis of depression. Her parents weren't together. Nor were Chantelle's, and her mother was depressed and possibly had an anxiety disorder, while her father was dependent on alcohol. No wonder the girls were angry; there was a lot to be angry about, and I said so.

'What do you mean?' Mo asked me.

'I mean there's a lot going on for all of you at home. You've all been through, and are still going through, lots of stuff, and it makes sense that you would feel angry about it.'

'My dad pisses me right off,' Saskia admitted. 'So does my mum for having him back every fucking time.'

'I can understand why,' I said, to validate her feelings.

'Can you?' she seemed surprised.

'Absolutely. And I'm also starting to understand why you might act in angry ways, sometimes, as a way to get some of that anger out. That goes for all of you, by the way, not just Saskia.'

'I think that might be why I wind people up,' Mo seemed pensive. 'I don't mean to, but it's like I can't help it. I just feel so wound up all the time, so I pick fights with people, because I'm just so full of... I don't know... this kind of *rage*.'

'Full of shit, more like,' Mercedes joked, and Mo smiled. 'Seriously though, I know what you mean. I think I do that sometimes as well.'

I knew what Mo and Mercedes meant too. As I've discussed elsewhere, they were describing the classic defence mechanism of displacement, which involves (unconsciously) taking a feeling response that belongs in one scenario and shifting it onto another. This is one of the ways that our mind (unconsciously) protects itself from becoming overwhelmed when we feel frightened, which would be an ordinary, appropriate response to being in a violent or threatening situation. Because violent and threatening situations were commonplace for the girls, they presented as if they had become desensitised to danger, and in a way, they had. I think that they tried to internalise the aggressive thoughts and impulses – that is, keep them to themselves – which is why they sometimes presented as withdrawn and dismissive. But when the thoughts and feelings became too much, they were acted outwards, in an attempt to get rid of them. Hence, the acts of anger and aggression I'd heard about and witnessed. I thought it might help the girls to think about this together, to use what can be framed as psychoeducation, which isn't therapy as such, but it can certainly feel reassuring (and therapeutic) for a young person who is beginning to make sense of the way they feel, think and behave.

I said, 'I think what Mo and Mercedes have said makes a lot of sense.'

'Me too,' Chantelle agreed. 'I think my mum does that. Takes it out on me when she's angry with my dad.'

'It's quite common,' I said, 'Especially when it feels too risky to get angry with the person that we're actually angry with.'

'So, like, if someone's being bullied, they go and pick on someone else who's weaker than them, rather than stand up to the bully?' Chantelle was really grappling to come to terms with the concept of displacement.

'Yes, that's the same sort of thing,' I assured her.

'So, rather than risk getting punched in the face by my dad if I tell him what a fucking cunt he is, I piss my boyfriend off, over nothing, because I know he'd never hit me?' Saskia was getting it too.

'Yes, that kind of thing too. So, when you get angry and rageful, seemingly for no apparent reason, there is absolutely a reason; it might just not be obvious what the reason is because it's about something that happened before or with someone else.'

'This shit makes a lot of sense,' Mercedes admitted.

'I'm pleased you think so.' I smiled. 'And that's why "this shit" is so interesting to me, because it makes sense of what's going on for *you* and demonstrates that how you act is saying something about how you feel.'

'So, you're saying it's not our fault?' Chantelle asked.

This was a tricky question. 'I'm saying that how we behave is a communication about how we feel and that it should be taken notice of, not just dismissed or punished,' I ventured. 'But also, as adults and young adults, we have to take responsibility for our actions, while accepting that we are in no way responsible for the things that happen to us growing up.' I think my response covered all the bases.

'Blame the parents!' Mo exclaimed.

'I'm not blaming parents, either,' I hastened to add, 'because there's a reason why *they* behave the way they do, too. We're simply trying to make sense of what's going on.'

Mo's statement, which was made half-jokingly, half-seriously, reminded me of the 1971 Philip Larkin poem 'This Be the Verse', which begins with the frequently quoted line, 'They fuck you up, your mum and dad…' But Larkin wasn't blaming parents either, and the poem continues, quite eloquently and astutely, to say, 'They may not mean to, but they do/They fill you with the faults they had/And add some extra, just for you/But they were fucked up in their turn/By fools in old-style hats and coats/Who half the time were soppy-stern/And half at one another's throats' (Larkin, 2003). Half a century ago, the poet was saying the same thing that psychoanalysts and psychotherapists have been saying since psychoanalysts and psychotherapists have been saying anything: that, while most parents are doing their best, most of the time, they too are shaped by what was going on during their own childhoods – hence the cross-generational repetition of experience, the stubbornly ingrained family scripts and the silhouettes of ghosts in the nursery (Fraiberg et al., 1975). What was going on for Chantelle, Mo, Mercedes, Connie and Saskia (and, I hypothesised, for many of their parents too) was physical and verbal domestic abuse, loss of a parent, emotional neglect, and experience of family members who were depressed, who misused drugs and alcohol and who were or had been in prison.

As I've already said, according to the research, there is a link between the number of ACEs experienced in childhood and negative physical and mental health outcomes in later life. Of particular interest is the research suggesting a causal link, rather than a mere correlation, between ACEs and antisocial behaviour (Fagan & Benedini, 2019), particularly when they occur in adolescence rather than in early childhood (Thornberry, et al., 2010). But I still believe in the potential for a better outcome for young people than the gloomy statistics or Larkin's poem would have us believe. I couldn't do what I do if I didn't.

One of the ways that change can happen, and it won't surprise you that I say this, is through the provision of loving, holding psychotherapy. According to research with young people who have experienced adversity, a central feature of a successful therapeutic intervention is the establishment of trust, not just in the therapeutic alliance, but through activities that build trust between peers (Oberle et al., 2016), such as group work. This is no mean feat, when young people have experienced multiple adversities and have a well-developed sense of mistrust. But by sticking with it and sticking with *them*, and by demonstrating a motivation to witness their boredom, anger and more 'without panicking or looking for a quick fix' (Luxmoore, 2019, p.46), adolescents can learn to trust us, the therapeutic process and themselves, and, through that process, change can happen.

10

F*cking nodding

Psychotherapists who work primarily with adolescents are warned against the 'hopeful notion' of a 'happy ever after' because to work with this age group is often to work 'on the border' (Waddell, 2018). What I think the esteemed child and adolescent psychotherapist Margot Waddell meant by this statement is that the period of adolescence is turbulent; the internal and external lives of adolescents are turbulent, and, by extension, therapy with adolescents, whether individual or in groups, is turbulent too. We find ourselves working at the edge of the relationship, the edge of therapy, the edge of the boundaries, the edge of risk and the edge of safeguarding. We find ourselves flip-flopping between feelings of love and hate and positions of trust and mistrust, because adolescents are flip-flopping too. This is why therapy with 16-year-olds is a tricky business. It's tempestuous and chaotic; sometimes it can provoke feelings of anger or boredom, and it's certainly not for everyone. It takes skill and pluck and can test the mettle of even the most experienced of therapists. As I said at the start of this book, and have illustrated throughout, being in the therapeutic space (both physically and metaphorically) with 16-year-olds is where anything can happen. It's the eye of the storm. It's demanding, challenging, intense and passionate. It's stimulating, entertaining and infuriating.

Some of the 16-year-olds who arrive in my therapy room feeling fragmented and 'all at sea' are keen to tell their stories; their thoughts and feelings spill out; they are unencumbered by self-consciousness; they are desperate to be heard and to be helped. Many are more reluctant to engage, and it takes time to build trust: in me, in the value of talking and listening and in themselves as narrators of their own experiences. They turn up tainted by past relationships with parents, peers and professionals. They don't speak, because experience has taught them that they won't be believed or listened to, or understood.

Or they talk non-stop to fill up the space and stop me from thinking. They feel exposed, so they try to hide. They feel vulnerable, so they lash out. They yearn for someone to get close enough to see the *real* them and understand the *real* them and love the *real* them, yet they push us and everyone else away. But there is always a reason to be hopeful and there is always potential for change. The fact that a young person has made it into my therapy room at all demonstrates that there is at least one small fibre of them that is hopeful and ready for change too. And that puts us on the same side, with the same common goal, no matter what they throw at me – verbally, literally or metaphorically – and that's worth remembering when the road gets rocky, which it often does with 16-year-olds, because they are almost certainly traversing a rocky road already.

In this book, I've shared some of my stories about psychotherapy with 16-year-olds. It's important to reiterate that these are *my* stories told from *my* perspective and influenced by *my* thinking and experiences. In order to understand what it's really like to be a 16-year-old in therapy, we'd have to ask a 16-year-old in therapy, and so it seems fitting that the last word should go to Mercedes, not least because she's a young person who likes having the last word. I asked her what she would say to a 16-year-old considering psychotherapy and she was quick to answer.

'Don't do it!'
'Really?'
'Yeah, really.'
'But you did it.'
'No, I didn't.'
'You did.'
'I dropped out.'
'You didn't drop out. We decided together that you might prefer the group to the one-to-one sessions. I don't see that as dropping out.'
'How do you see it, then?'
'I think maybe we got it wrong at first.'
'*You* got it wrong?'
'Yes. I think maybe we shouldn't have suggested individual psychotherapy for you. Sometimes adults get it wrong.'
'They don't usually admit it though. But you're not a usual kind of adult.'
'I'm not sure how to take that...'

'It's a compliment.'
'Well in that case, thank you.'
'You're welcome. Thank you, too.'
'What for?'
'For this. For bothering with me.'
'You're welcome. Thank *you* for bothering to give it a go.'
'It wasn't so bad, in the end. I quite liked the group.'
'I think the group quite liked you too.' I smiled and Mercedes smiled because we knew it was true and that it's nice to feel liked.
'I wonder what it was that you liked or found helpful?'
'I think just knowing there were other people who'd fucked up like me and listening to each other's stories and, you know, just being there for each other.'
'I agree. I think listening and being there for someone are underrated qualities.'
'Yeah. I suppose that pretty much describes your day job.'
'Pretty much.'
'Cool.'
'So, thinking about this imaginary 16-year-old who's thinking about starting therapy with an imaginary therapist…'
'What about them?'
'What would you say to them about what to expect?'
'You rock up and you tell someone everything about how you think and feel, and everything about what you do and all the stuff you never thought you'd tell anyone…'
'But only when you're ready and only if you want to…' I was a bit alarmed.
'Yeah, that's true, but I didn't know that at first. I thought you *had* to.'
'So maybe you could tell them that – that while you might think you have to tell all, it's up to you what you talk about and when and even if you say anything at all?'
'Yeah, I'd tell them that.'
'Good. I think that would be helpful.'
'Okay. I'll make sure to tell Little Miss Imaginary Sixteen-Year-Old.'
'Great. And what about what the therapist does while you're telling all, or not telling all, or whatever you've decided to tell?'
'She stays shtum and tells you absolutely fucking nothing about herself or her own life, which is fucking *rude*!'

'How is it rude?'

'Well, it's not really rude. It seems rude at first, like it's all one-sided, but then you get used to it and you get it.'

'What do you get?'

'That they're "there for you".' Mercedes made air quotes around 'there for you'.

'So, then it feels okay that the therapist doesn't talk about themselves?'

'Yeah. Absolutely. It's not about them, it's about you!'

'Absolutely! Anything else you'd say?'

'That therapy is weird.'

'I agree.'

'You're a therapist!'

'I am, but I agree that what happens in therapy is quite unlike what happens out there, in the real world…'

'Yeah. Talking about yourself for 50 minutes while someone else just sits there listening and nodding is weird.'

'Fucking nodding?' I asked, taking up the position of the barely-there smile, sympathetic eyes and gently nodding my head.

'Yeah, fucking nodding!'

References

American Psychiatric Association. (2013). *The diagnostic and statistical manual of mental disorders (DSM)* (5th ed.). American Psychiatric Association.

Asmussen, K., Fischer, F., Drayton, E. & McBride, T. (2020). *What we know, what we don't know, and what should happen next*. Early Intervention Foundation.

Bartholomew, K. & Horowitz, L.M. (1991). Attachment styles among young adults: A test of a four-category model. *Journal of Personality and Social Psychology, 61*(2), 226–244.

Bergson, H. (1983). *Creative evolution* (A. Mitchell, trans.). University Press of America. (First published in French 1907).

Bick, E. (1968). The experience of the skin in early object relations. *International Journal of Psychoanalysis, 49*(2–3), 484–486.

Bion, W.R. (1961). *Experiences in groups and other papers*. Routledge.

Bion, W.R. (1962). *Learning from experience*. Heinemann.

Bowlby, J. (1979). *The making and breaking of affectional bonds*. Taylor & Francis.

Brazelton, T.B. & Cramer, B.G. (1990). *The earliest relationship: Parents, infants and the drama of early attachment*. Da Capo Press.

Byng-Hall, J. (1995). *Rewriting family scripts: Improvisation and systems change*. Guilford Press.

Cambridge Dictionary (2021). Fetish. [Online.] https://dictionary.cambridge.org/dictionary/english/fetish

Canham, H. (2002). Group and gang states of mind. *Journal of Child Psychotherapy, 28*(2), 113–129.

Coltart, N. (1993). *Slouching towards Bethlehem*. Free Association Books.

Connor, J. (2020). *Reflective practice in child and adolescent psychotherapy: Listening to young people*. Routledge.

Crown Prosecution Service. (2020). *Therapy: Provision of therapy for child witnesses prior to a criminal trial*. [Online.] www.cps.gov.uk/legal-guidance/therapy-provision-therapy-child-witnesses-prior-criminal-trial

Elson, M. (1986). *Self-psychology in clinical social work*. W.W. Norton & Co.

Fagan, A.A. & Benedini, K.M. (2019). Family influences on youth offending. In D.P. Farrington, L. Kazemian & A.R. Piquero (Eds.), *The Oxford handbook of developmental and life-course criminology* (pp.378–403). Oxford University Press.

Fox, C. & Hawton, K. (2004). *Deliberate self-harm in adolescence*. Jessica Kingsley Publishers.

Fraiberg, S., Adelson, E. & Shapiro, V. (1975) Ghosts in the nursery: A psychoanalytic approach to the problems of impaired infant-mother relationships. *Journal of American Academy of Child Psychiatry, 14*(3), 387–421.

Freud, A. (1937). *The ego and the mechanisms of defence*. Hogarth Press/Institute of Psychoanalysis.

Freud, S. (1896/2001). The aetiology of hysteria. In *The standard edition of the complete psychological works of Sigmund Freud. Vol. 3.* (J. Strachey, trans.). Vintage.

Freud, S. (1905/2001). Three essays on the theory of sexuality. In *The standard edition of the complete psychological works of Sigmund Freud. Vol 7.* (J. Strachey, trans.). Vintage.

Freud, S. (1909/2001). Notes upon a case of obsessional neurosis (Der Rattenmann). In *The standard edition of the complete psychological works of Sigmund Freud. Vol. 10.* (J. Strachey, trans.). Vintage.

Freud, S. (1910/2001). The origin and development of psychoanalysis. *American Journal of Psychology, 21*, 181–218.

Freud, S. (1917/2001) *Mourning and melancholia*. In The standard edition of the complete psychological works of Sigmund Freud. Vol. 14. (J. Strachey, trans.). Vintage.

Freud, S. (1920/2001). Beyond the pleasure principle. In *The standard edition of the complete psychological works of Sigmund Freud. Vol 18.* (J. Strachey, trans.). Vintage.

Freud, S. (1921/2001). *Group psychology and the analysis of the ego*. In The standard edition of the complete psychological works of Sigmund Freud. Vol. 13. (J. Strachey, trans.). Vintage.

Freud Museum. (2018). *Gradiva: The cure through love*. [Online.] www.freud.org.uk/exhibitions/gradiva/

Gray, A. (2014). *An introduction to the therapeutic frame*. Routledge. (First published 1994).

Hinshelwood, R. & Skogstad, W. (2000) *Observing organisations: Anxiety, defence and culture in health care*. Routledge.

Holleb, M.L.E. (2019). *The A–Z of gender and sexuality: From Ace to Ze*. Jessica Kingsley Publishers.

Jennings, S. (1998) *Introduction to dramatherapy*. Jessica Kingsley Publishers.

Jennings, S. (2011). *Healthy attachments and neuro-dramatic play*. Jessica Kingsley Publishers.

Johnstone, L. (2022). *A straight talking introduction to psychiatric diagnosis* (2nd ed.). PCCS Books.

Jung, C.G. (1968). *The archetypes and the collective unconscious*. Routledge.

Kahn, L. (2017). *Baffled by love: Stories of the lasting impact of childhood trauma inflicted by loved ones*. She Writes Press.

Kantrowitz, J.L. (2020). *The role of the patient-analyst match in the process and outcome of psychoanalysis*. Routledge.

Kazdin, A.E. (1990). Psychotherapy for children and adolescents. *Annual Review of Psychology, 41*, 21–54.

Kegerreis, S. (1993). From a gang of two back to the family. *Psychoanalytic Psychotherapy, 7*(1), 69–83.

Kegerreis, S. (2010). *Psychodynamic counselling with children and young people*. Palgrave Macmillan.

Klein, M. (1932). *The psychoanalysis of children*. Hogarth Press.

Klein, M. (1957). *Envy and gratitude: A study of unconscious sources*. Tavistock Publications.

Kohut, H. (1959). Introspection, empathy, and psychoanalysis: An examination of the relationship between mode of observation and theory. *Journal of the American Psychoanalytic Association, 7*, 459–483.

Kohut, H. (1971). *The analysis of the self: A systematic approach to the psychoanalytic treatment of narcissistic personality disorders*. International Universities Press.

Laufer, M. & Laufer, M.E. (1995). *Adolescence and developmental breakdown: A psychoanalytical view*. Karnac Books.

Larkin, P. (2003). This be the verse. In *Collected Poems*. Faber & Faber.

Lawrence, W.G. (1977). Management development: Some ideals, images and realities. In A.D. Colman & M.H. Gelle, *Group relations reader 2*. A.K. Rice Institute.

Luxmoore, N. (2010). *Young people in love and hate*. Jessica Kingsley Publishers.

Luxmoore, N. (2019). *The art of working with anxious, antagonistic adolescents: Ways forward for frontline professionals*. Jessica Kingsley Publishers.

McDougall, J. (1995). *The many faces of Eros*. Free Association Books.

Mellier, D. (2014). The psychic envelopes in psychoanalytic theories of infancy. *Frontiers in Psychology 5*, 734. doi:10.3389/fpsyg.2014.00734

Milner, M. (1952). Aspects of symbolisms and comprehension of the not-self. *International Journal of Psychoanalysis 33*, 181–195.

Moncrieff, J. (2020). *A straight talking introduction to psychiatric drugs* (2nd ed.). PCCS Books.

Nagel T. (1974) What is it like to be a bat? *The Philosophical Review, 83*(4), 435–450.

National Institute on Drug Abuse (NIDA). (2011). *Real teens ask: Is addiction hereditary?* [Online.] https://archives.drugabuse.gov/blog/post/real-teens-ask-addiction-hereditary

National and Specialist OCD, BDD and Related Disorders Service for Young People, Maudsley Hospital. (2019). *Appearance anxiety.* Jessica Kingsley Publishers.

NHS (2019). *Symptoms of clinical depression.* [Online.] www.nhs.uk/mental-health/conditions/clinical-depression/symptoms/

NHS (2020). *Body dysmorphic disoprder (BDD).* [Online.] www.nhs.uk/mental-health/conditions/body-dysmorphia/

Oberle, E., Domitrovich, C.E., Meyers, D.C. & Weissberg, R.P. (2016). Establishing systemic social and emotional learning approaches in schools: A framework for schoolwide implementation. *Cambridge Journal of Education, 46*(3), 277–297.

Office of the High Commissioner for Human Rights (OHCHR). *The convention on the rights of the child.* United Nations. www.ohchr.org/en/professionalinterest/pages/crc.aspx?fbclid=IwAR35cVUouzhmgWieqVBgZYcB2B0AxOmow0WCMu4zy7eIWfQD-VMAwGkORks.

O'Keane, V. (2021). *The rag and bone shop: How we make memories and how memories make us.* Allen Lane.

Orbach, S. (2009). *Bodies.* Profile Books.

Oxford English Dictionary. (2021). *Love.* www.oed.com/viewdictionaryentry/Entry/110566.

Parker, G. & Eyers, K. (2010). *Navigating teenage depression: A guide for parents and professionals.* Routledge.

Redland, D. (2020). *Psychoanalytic perspectives on women, menstruation and secondary amenorrhea.* Routledge.

Reid, S. (1999). The group as a healing whole: Group psychotherapy with children and adolescents. In M. Lanyado & A. Horne, *The handbook of child psychotherapy* (pp.247–259). Routledge.

Roberts, V.Z. (1994). The self-assigned impossible task. In A. Obholzer & V.Z. Roberts (Eds.), *The unconscious at work: Individual and organisational stress in the human services* (pp.110–119). Routledge.

Roche, J. (2020). *Gender explorers.* Jessica Kingsley Publishers.

Rogers, C.R. (1961). *On becoming a person: A psychotherapist's view of psychotherapy.* Houghton Mifflin.

Rosen, M. (1993). *We're going on a bear hunt.* Walker Books.

Royal College of Psychiatrists (2021). *Depression in children and young people: for young people.* [Online.] www.rcpsych.ac.uk/mental-health/parents-and-young-people/young-people/depression-in-children-and-young-people-for-young-people

Salzberger-Wittenberg, I. (1970). Phantasy. In *Psychanalytic insights and relationships: A Kleinian approach* (pp.20–30). Brunner-Routledge.

School of Sexuality Education. (2021). *Sex Ed: An inclusive teenage guide to sex and relationships*. Walker Books.

Simon, R. (2020). *The every body book*. Jessica Kingsley Publishers.

Soper, C.A. (2018). *The evolution of suicide*. Springer.

Steinem, G. (2019). *The truth will set you free, but first it will piss you off!* Murdoch Books.

Stokes, J. (1994). The unconscious at work in groups and teams: Contributions from the work of Wilfred Bion. In Obholzer, A. & Roberts V.Z. (Eds.), *The unconscious at work: Individual and organisational stress in the human services* (pp.19–27). Routledge.

Suttie, I.D. (1935). *The origins of love and hate*. Routledge, Trench, Trubner & Co.

Thornberry, T.P., Henry, K.L., Ireland, T.O. & Smith, C.A. (2010). The causal impact of childhood-limited maltreatment and adolescent maltreatment on early adult adjustment. *Journal of Adolescent Health, 46*(4), 359–365.

Timimi, S. (2021). *A straight talking introduction to children's mental health problems* (2nd ed.). PCCS Books.

Vaillant, G. (1994). Ego mechanisms of defence and personality psychopathology. *Journal of Abnormal Psychology, 103*(1), 44–50.

Van Buskirk, W. & McGrath, D. (1999). Organisational cultures as holding environments: A psychodynamic look at organisational symbolism. *Human Relations, 52*(6), 805–832.

Very Well Mind. (2019). Cognitive developmental milestones. [Online.] www.verywellmind.com/cognitive-developmental-milestones-2795109#from-2-to-3-years

Waddell, M. (2018). *On adolescence: Inside stories*. The Tavistock Clinic Series. Karnac.

Watson, J. (2019a). There's an intruder in our house! Counselling, psychotherapy and the biomedical model of emotional distress. In J. Watson (Ed.), *Drop the disorder! Challenging the culture of psychiatric diagnosis* (pp.223–237). PCCS Books.

Watson, J. (Ed.) (2019b). *Drop the disorder! Challenging the culture of psychiatric diagnosis*. PCCS Books.

Whitely, M., Raven, M., Timimi, S., Jureidini, J., Phillimore, J., Leo, J., Moncrieff, J. & Landman, P. (2018). ADHD late birthdate effect common in both high and low prescribing international jurisdictions: Systematic review. *Journal of Child Psychology and Psychiatry, 60*(4), 380–391.

Williams, G. (1997). *Internal landscapes and foreign bodies: Eating disorders and other pathologies*. Karnac.

Williams, J. (1997). *Cry of pain: Understanding suicide and self-harm*. Penguin Books.

Windust, J. (2021). *In their shoes: Navigating non-binary life*. Jessica Kingsley Publishers.

Winnicott, D.W. (1965a). Ego distortion in terms of true and false self. In *The maturational process and the facilitating environment: Studies in the theory of emotional development* (pp.140-152). Hogarth Press.

Winnicott, D.W. (1965b). *The maturational process and the facilitating environment: Studies in the theory of emotional development*. Hogarth Press.

Winnicott, D.W. (1986a). *Home is where we start from: Essays by a psychoanalyst*. C. Winnicott, R. Shepherd, & M. Davis (Eds.). Penguin Books.

Winnicott, D.W. (1986b). Delinquency as a sign of hope. In C. Winnicott, R. Shepherd & M. Davis (Eds.), *Home is where we start from: Essays by a psychoanalyst* (pp.90-100). Penguin Books.

Wright, B., Garside, M., Allgar, V., Hodkinson, R. & Thorpe, H. (2020). A large population-based study of the mental health and wellbeing of children and young people in the North of England. *Clinical Child Psychology and Psychiatry, 25*(4). doi.org/10.1177/1359104520925873

Name index

A
American Psychiatric Association (APA) 9
Asmussen, K. 185–186

B
Balint, M. 163
Bartholomew, K. 55
Benedini, K.M. 190
Bergson, H. 121
Bick, E. 163–164
Bion, W.R. 13, 18, 22, 23, 24, 28, 30, 31, 68, 77, 153, 183, 185
Bowlby, J. 13, 55
Brazelton, T.B. 49, 54, 166, 169
British Institute of Psychoanalysis 156
Byng-Hall, J. 58, 151

C
Cambridge Dictionary 109
Child and Adolescent Mental Health Services (CAMHS) 37, 103
Canham, H. 26
Coltart, N. 183
Connor, J. 12
Cramer, B.G. 49, 54, 166, 169
Crown Prosecution Service 40

E
Elson, M. 3
Eyers, K. 162, 168

F
Fagan, A.A. 190
Ferenczi 183
Fox, C. 91, 156

F
Fraiberg, S. 58, 140, 143, 166, 190
Freud, A. 156, 161
Freud, S. 5, 13, 57, 68, 82, 92, 100, 109, 111, 113, 147, 152, 161, 166, 183
Freud Museum 183

G
Gendered Intelligence 81
Gray, A. 8, 10, 24, 49, 50, 62, 170, 182, 183

H
Hawton, K. 91, 156
Hinshelwood, R. 23–24, 26
Holleb, M.L.E. 82, 90, 95
Horowitz, L.M. 55

J
Jennings, S. 182, 184
Johnstone, L. 10, 11
Jung, C.G. 98

K
Kahn, L. 135
Kantrowitz, J.L. 8
Kazdin, A.E. 6–7
Kegerreis, S. 26, 33, 152
Klein, M. 13, 43, 55, 90, 163, 180–181
Kohut, H. 3, 5, 100

L
Larkin, P. 13, 190
Laufer, M. 156–157, 165, 167
Laufer, M.E. 156–157, 165, 167

Lawrence, W.G. 18
Luxmoore, N. 178, 179, 183, 191

M
McDougall, J. 112
McGrath, D. 22-23, 145
Mellier, D. 164
Milner, M. 44
Moncrieff, J. 10

N
Nagel, T. 4-5
National Institute on Drug Abuse 112
National and Specialist OCD, BDD and Related Disorders Service for Young People, Maudsley Hospital 134
NHS 127, 134

O
Oberle, E. 191
Office of the High Commissioner for Human Rights (OHCHR) 1
O'Keane, V. 132
Orbach, S 13, 133, 135
Oxford English Dictionary 182

P
Parker, G. 162, 168

R
Redland, D. 60
Reid, S. 183
Roberts, V.Z. 23, 27, 28, 184
Roche, J. 83
Rogers, C.R. 181
Rosen, M. 13, 185
Royal College of Psychiatrists (RCPsych) 16-17

S
Salzberger-Wittenberg, I. 43, 55, 146
School of Sexuality Education 96
Simon, R. 96
Skogstad, W. 23-24, 26
Soper, C.A. 162

Steinem, G. 13, 136
Stokes, J. 24
Suttie, I.D. 183

T
Tavistock Clinic 163
Thornberry, T.P. 190
Timimi, S. 9, 10
TransActual 81

V
Vaillant, G. 99, 146
Van Buskirk, W. 22-23, 145
Very Well Mind 129

W
Waddell, M. 151, 180, 192
Watson, J. 10, 11
Whiteley, M. 129
Williams, G. 68, 135, 152, 168
Williams, J. 90, 156, 165
Windust, J. 85
Winnicott, D.W. 13, 31, 34, 100, 152, 182
Wright, B. 2

Subject index

A

abandonment 112, 114, 117, 143, 181
ACEs 135, 185–186, 190,
acting out 61, 77, 89, 146, 151–152, 171
addictive behaviour 111–113, 120
alcohol 7, 14, 59, 61, 64, 103, 112, 186, 188, 190
alpha function 68, 77
ambivalence 65, 82, 92, 101, 153, 180
anger 103, 106, 116, 149, 186, 188–189, 190, 192
   management 13, 103, 106–108, 119–120, 176
antisocial behaviour 152, 190
anxiety 11, 15, 23, 25, 27–28, 35, 37–38, 56, 78, 82, 92, 112, 133, 161, 166, 184
assessment 9, 61–62, 64–65, 126, 161–162
attachment 13, 55, 157, 182
attention deficit hyperactivity disorder (ADHD) 9, 129
authentic self (*see also* true self) 7 8, 101

B

behaviour 6–7, 9, 37, 43–44, 61, 85, 121, 129, 132, 134, 180–181
   anti-social, 137–138, 144, 149, 151–152,
   attention-seeking, 90, 98, 155
   eating, 25, 121–122, 131–132
   risky, 7, 61, 71, 77, 132,
   sexual, 61, 69–73, 107–120
   suicidal, 155–156, 165–166, 179
being seen 42, 44, 47, 53, 104, 133, 163
body 68, 78, 84, 86–90, 94, 98, 109, 131–132, 157, 163
   body dysmorphia 121, 133
   body image 131
boundaries
   sexual, 66, 73,
   therapeutic, 22, 44, 49–50, 54, 59, 82, 93, 190, 182–183, 192

C

child in care (*see also* looked after child) 102, 104
colour-
   blind 104
   conscious 104
competition 24, 135
compulsion 88, 102, 112–113, 115, 119, 166
confidentiality 22, 38, 45, 52, 90, 99, 183
consultation 36, 38–39, 43, 55, 57, 78, 82, 85, 99, 121, 124, 134, 138, 153, 165
container 22, 28, 68, 76, 164, 182, 184
containment (*see also* holding) 50, 68, 145, 164
content 3, 47–49, 56, 89
countertransference 8, 23–24, 138, 152

D

deadname 100
defence (*see also* denial, displacement, projection, second skin, splitting, sublimation) 2, 27,

92, 99, 117, 147, 160–161, 166–167, 171, 188
denial 12, 159–160
depression 17, 37, 78, 103, 123–124, 126–127, 133–134, 162, 166–167, 171
diagnosing 7, 9–11
disavow 26, 111, 113
displacement 188–189
domestic abuse 143, 188, 190

E

eating disorder 121–122, 132, 134
ending 56, 77, 117–118
enmeshment 68
envy 135
erotic transference 8, 108–109
ethical dilemma 40, 89, 91
ethnicity (race) 54, 90, 10–106

F

false self 100
family 3, 30–31, 34, 43, 49, 59–62, 81, 90, 159, 165, 186
   history 5, 36, 103, 112–113, 139,
   script 58, 84, 171, 190
   secret 57, 153
fantasy 22, 43, 57, 130, 143, 145–147, 171
fathers 31–32, 42, 56, 58, 59, 62, 68–69, 76, 84, 103, 112, 139, 142–145, 150, 152, 158, 165, 188
fetish 102, 105–113, 118–119
first sessions 20, 47, 57, 59, 62, 82, 89, 172
first sex 71–73
formulation 10–11, 79, 105
fragmentation/fragmented 3, 100–101, 181, 192

G

gang(s) 25–26, 137–138, 139, 151–153, 180
gender 78, 81–84, 90, 92, 94–96, 101
   dysphoria 90, 96

identity 83, 95
ghosts in the nursery 58, 142–144, 146, 166, 171, 190
good enough 15, 22, 28, 35
   mother/parent 55, 68, 116, 119–120, 121, 153, 164, 181
   therapist/therapy 23, 55, 116
group
   process 22–23, 31, 185,
   task 22, 183
   work 15, 17, 23, 172, 183, 191

H

here and now 3, 5, 8, 24, 31, 82, 150, 180
humour 20, 98
hypothesis 3, 43, 48, 54, 61, 76, 79, 92, 105, 113, 156, 166

I

identity 12, 18, 25, 34, 83–84, 95
infant observation 163, 168
initial consultation 36, 38, 43, 57, 78, 85, 121, 134, 138, 153
integration (*see also* reintegration) 3, 85
intellectualise 112, 119
intimacy 14, 47, 55, 63, 105, 119

L

labelling 10–12, 80, 83, 97, 111, 126–127, 133–134
lateness 28, 48, 82, 93
LGBTQA+ 85
looked after child (*see also:* child in care) 104
loss 34, 113, 152, 159, 165, 190
low mood 15, 122, 127, 133

M

masturbation (*see also* wanking) 95, 98, 99, 106, 114
maternal 118
   attachment 182
   containment 164

transference 114, 119
menstruation 88, 133, 135
metaphor (*see also* symbolic/symbolism) 22, 144–145, 148, 149, 192
minimising 133, 140, 144, 155, 156, 158, 160
misgender 81
mothers (*see also* good-enough mother) 13, 33, 54, 55, 58, 62, 103, 112–116, 119–120, 141, 143, 146, 152, 154, 156, 165, 170–171, 180, 182, 188

N

normalising 3, 133, 152
not-knowing 22, 38, 52, 57, 92, 100, 178

O

Oedipus 152
online therapy 45
outcome measures (*see also* quantitative assessment) 37, 161

P

pansexual 95
projection 91–92, 100, 146–147, 155, 165, 184
pseudo independence 164–165, 171
psychoanalytic (*see also* psychodynamic) 5, 13, 68, 101, 112, 113, 134, 156, 160, 164–166, 180, 183
psychodynamic (*see also* psychoanalytic) 1, 3–5, 8, 13, 23–24, 26–27, 68, 92, 99, 112, 152, 156, 166
psychoeducation 11, 186, 189
puberty 2, 12, 83, 87, 132, 134, 151, 156, 180

Q

quantitative assessment (*see also* outcome measures) 37, 161

R

reintegration (*see also* integration) 100–101
rejection 102, 117, 160, 181
reparation 34, 120, 134
repetition compulsion 57, 82, 113, 115, 142
rivalry 24, 135

S

safeguarding 70, 89, 138, 192
school refusal 127, 133
second skin 163–164, 166, 171
secrets 43, 57
self, sense of 2–3, 55, 59, 62, 66, 84, 100, 121, 132, 135, 172, 180
self-esteem 15–17, 121–122, 134–135
self-injury 15, 64, 68, 80, 86, 89–91, 101
self-loathing 87, 89
self-soothing 98, 113
separation 31, 180, 186
sex 60–61, 66, 69, 71–74, 87, 94–98, 109, 115, 132, 141, 185
  education 87, 95, 96
sexuality 78, 81, 83, 95, 101, 111, 118, 133, 135
social withdrawal 127, 133
splitting 63, 115, 147
sublimation 92, 99
suicidal 1, 124, 127, 132–134, 155–156, 165–167, 171
symbolic/symbolism (*see also* metaphor) 24, 44, 62, 68, 76, 86, 98, 100, 109, 113, 118, 136, 144, 170, 183

T

therapeutic
  frame 44, 50, 183
  process 6, 23, 30–31, 47–48, 49, 56, 91, 99, 133, 169, 191
  relationship 3, 8, 43–44, 65, 77, 91, 101, 105, 134, 180, 182–183
therapy review 37, 55, 127

transference (*see also* erotic
    transference, maternal
    transference) 3, 8–9, 17, 24,
    60, 67, 108, 114–115, 117,
    119
transgender 80, 82, 85, 94–95
transition 2, 12, 26, 78, 83, 87, 110,
    135, 151
trauma 131, 135, 143, 181
true self (*see also* authentic self) 100

U
unconscious 3–4, 13, 22, 68, 98, 101,
    112–113, 120, 138, 143, 147,
    152, 166, 171, 184

W
wanking (*see also* masturbation)
    96–97, 105–106, 107, 116,
    120
withholding 38–39, 43, 46, 50, 57, 106,
    119, 122, 181